Lamaze is for Chickens

A Guide to Prepared Childbirth

Mimi Green
Maxine Naab

Cartoons
by
Pamela Tapia

AVERY PUBLISHING GROUP INC.
Wayne, New Jersey

Permission Credits

Figure 2.5: Adapted from Garrey et al., *Obstetrics Illustrated,* Third Edition: Churchill Livingstone, 1980, Edinburgh.

Figures 2.7 and 2.8: From "The Topographic History of the Volar Pads (Walking Pads; Tastballen) in the Human Embryo," by Harold Cummins, in *Contributions to Embryology*. Reprinted by permission of the publisher, Carnegie Institution of Washington.

Figure 2.9: Reprinted with permission of Ross Laboratories, Columbus, OH 43216. From Mechanism of Normal Labor, Clinical Education Aid No. 13, © 1979 Ross Laboratories.

Figures 4.1 and 4.3: Reprinted with permission of Ross Laboratories, Columbus, OH 43216. From Obstetrical Presentation and Position, Clinical Education Aid No. 18, © 1978 Ross Laboratories.

The authors and publisher would like to thank John A. Bohrer, Brenda Lynn Friese, and Diane Wilson for allowing us to reproduce photos of their births. We also thank Mary Jo McKenna for allowing us to reproduce the chapter "Here We Go Again."

Library of Congress Cataloging-in-Publication Data
Green, Mimi.
Lamaze is for chickens.

(Avery childbirth education series)
Bibliography: p.
Includes index.
1. Natural childbirth. 2. Infants--Care and hygiene. I. Naab, Maxine. II. Title. III. Series.
[DNLM: 1. Infant Care--popular works. 2. Natural Childbirth. 3. Pregnancy--popular works. WQ 150 G7971]
RG661.G74 1985 618.4'5 85-11146
ISBN 0-89529-181-9 (pbk.)

Cover Design: Martin Hochberg and Rudy Shur
Cover Art: Pamela Tapia
Cover Art Separations: Tim Peterson
In-House Editor: Joanne Abrams

Printed in the United States of America

10 9 8 7 6 5 4 3 2 1

Contents

What Lamaze Is • Pain Is a Part of Life • A Word to Fathers • The History of Childbirth Preparation • Dealing With Pain in Labor: The Lamaze Techniques

Maternal Anatomy • Fetal Anatomy • Physical Changes During Pregnancy • Exercises • Preparing for Childbirth

Labor Begins • What to Take to the Hospital • Hospital Admission Routines • The Physical Process of Childbirth • The Postpartum Period • The Emotional Aspects of Childbirth

Dedication

This manual is fondly dedicated to those doctors who have given us so much support and encouragement; to the nurses who lovingly care for our students during childbirth; and to the couples who thought they could not do it, but who did it anyway. Their joy in the birth of their babies has made teaching these classes an extremely satisfying experience.

Acknowledgements

The material in this book was developed through research as well as through our own personal experiences in labor and the experiences of the couples we have trained. We sincerely wish to thank Dr. Daniel Bohi and Karen Green, R.N., for their encouragement and assistance in the preparation of the original manual. David Chamberlain designed the superb illustrations of the baby *in utero*. We greatly appreciate his skill and help. We also thank Rose Chamberlain, who typed and edited the original manuscript in preparation for printing.

Special thanks go to Mary Jo McKenna, a valued friend and excellent childbirth educator, for her support and encouragement throughout the writing of this revised edition. Mary Jo also contributed the excellent chapter "Here We Go Again," about the specific concerns of families expecting another baby.

Many helped in the preparation of this revised edition, but we especially want to thank Dr. Charles Marlowe and Kathy Hensley for their helpful comments and suggestions. Our most grateful thanks go to Barbara Glazeski, who read and critiqued the final edition.

Preface

Now that you are pregnant, you may notice things that you never saw before. There are expectant couples everywhere; conversation always gravitates toward a discussion of pregnancy and labor, even if you began discussing the merits of yogurt over sour cream in a particular recipe; there are many sales on baby items, and you just missed another one; and books on pregnancy, baby names, birth, and parenting appear suddenly in every aisle of the grocery store. Well, here is yet another of those books on childbirth, but this is the best one! Because these topics are important to you now, we have chosen to thoroughly cover pregnancy, childbirth, and some aspects of life with a baby. We have included discussions of the do's and don'ts of pregnancy, prenatal exercises, and fetal development. The topics of adjusting to a new baby, infant nutrition, and birth control are also covered. The most detailed coverage has been given to the Lamaze form of prepared childbirth.

The term "birth attendant" is used frequently throughout the text, and may need some clarification. Today, people of many different backgrounds are available to assist parents during the birth of their baby. For consistency and clarity, we have used the term "birth attendant" when referring to the physician or midwife. All pronouns referring to the physician, midwife, or baby are "he" or "him." Of course your doctor or midwife may be a woman, and your baby may be

Christina instead of Christopher. We hope that no one will be offended by our use of the male pronouns.

While we are clarifying terms, here is another. We have used the term "birthing area" to refer to the place that you have chosen as your birth environment. Most of you have probably chosen to go to a hospital, but other options, such as alternate birthing centers, are available in many localities.

Although the terms of this manual apply primarily to married couples, you will still benefit from Lamaze preparation and from this text if you are single. The same information applies whether or not the person with whom you are sharing this experience is the father of your baby. If you have a continuing relationship with your child's father, he will be a good partner or labor coach. However, if this is not possible, anyone who cares for you and is interested in working with you will be just as helpful.

It is our fervent wish that you will enjoy the birth of your baby and that this manual will be instrumental in that momentous event in your life. Read it and learn what labor and birth can be like. Practice the exercises for labor and birth, and use them to the best of your ability during your own labor. Read the sections on early parenting before your baby's birth, so you will be familiar with the variety of emotions that parents may experience during the early months, and know that you are not alone. Keep this section handy for easy reference after your baby arrives.

Birth can be one of the most rewarding experiences of your life, and being a parent is one of life's greatest challenges. We hope that this manual will help you prepare for both.

Chapter One
Get Ready

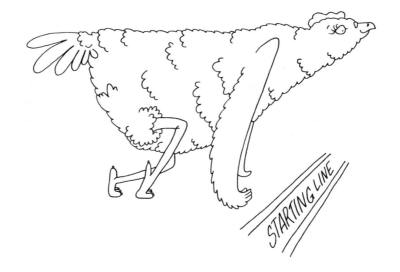

STARTING LINE

WHAT LAMAZE IS

If you are not well acquainted with Lamaze childbirth—which is also called the Psychoprophylactic Method of Preparation for Childbirth—you may not believe the title of this book. You may have heard that Lamaze is "natural" childbirth, which may suggest that you discretely disappear behind a bush, deliver your baby, strap him to your back, and resume your work in the field. Nothing special has happened. Birth is just part of another day's work.

Fortunately for us chickens (those of us who are afraid of pain) Lamaze is not "natural" childbirth. The breathing, concentration, and relaxation techniques you will use in labor are all learned skills. For an unprepared woman in our society, "natural" birth is improbable. A dog needs no preparation to give birth "naturally." But then nobody told her how much it hurts to have a puppy. We are victims of our culture. Years ago, whenever women had long, difficult labors, everyone heard all the unpleasant details. No one heard about the easy labors, because they did not make good stories. When gas (ether, in 1846, and later chloroform) was first used for childbirth, women everywhere rejoiced. Finally, there was no need to fear a painful birth. The woman went

1

to the hospital, was given a drug to induce sleep, and awakened several hours after her baby's birth to be told that she was the mother of a boy or girl. She had some vomiting, her baby was very sleepy, and for several years she had vague recollections of severe pain. But during each labor she could again be removed from the situation. Unfortunately, some mothers reacted adversely to the inhalation anesthesia, and some babies took much too long to begin breathing.

Further advances have been made in obstetrics, and today there is no reason to fear childbirth. But many still do. Vivid impressions of difficult labors received from well-meaning friends and relatives are hard to erase. Because of these impressions, you may have thought that your friend who planned to have a Lamaze birth was crazy. But she had her baby, and said that the labor was okay and the delivery was great! Now you think that perhaps she can't feel pain, or that she was lucky this time. But in the back of your mind you hope she found something that will help you too. She did. Lamaze preparation will help you during labor and provide you with the satisfying experience of giving birth to your baby in a fearless and relaxed manner.

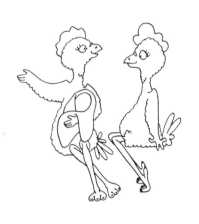

Lamaze is prepared childbirth. Nothing is left to chance. You will be taught to deal effectively with the sensations of your contractions. Lamaze is not unattended or unmedicated birth. A dedicated and efficient nursing staff and your chosen birth attendant will assist you in labor. Best of all, a person who cares a great deal about you—your husband, a close friend, or a relative—will be your labor partner.

Lamaze is not a leap backwards into the dark ages. This technique takes advantage of the modern advances in obstetrical care, and then goes further to fulfill some of the emotional and psychological needs of the expectant parents. The goal of your Lamaze training is not an unmedicated birth, or a birth without medical intervention, but a birth that will allow you to most fully experience the excitement and joy of the event.

Joy? Yes! Childbirth is a joyous time. Having a baby is one of life's peak experiences.

We say that childbirth is joyous and beautiful, but if you think that it will be painful, you may not believe that you will enjoy it. How can you enjoy childbirth when it is so painful? If you did not know how to swim, you might wonder how people could enjoy swimming. Not knowing how to swim might make you afraid of the ocean. In the ocean the waves would knock you over, water would flood your nose, and you would come up choking. Swimming—yuck! But if you knew how to swim you would float over the waves and really enjoy the challenge of mastering the ocean.

Suppose we tell you that on a certain date, someone will throw you into the ocean for several hours. Some of you who do not know how to swim will learn how to ahead of time. Others will await the day in terror, praying for a quick rescue. Those who will not learn to swim will know that they will be helped, but will not know how much they will have to suffer before being rescued. Every pregnant woman has her day in the ocean. Labor is that day. Some prepare, while others dread and pray.

Lamaze childbirth, like swimming, is a learned skill, requiring preparation. An infant has all the motor coordination necessary to swim, and has no fear of water. As he grows older, he learns to fear water and "forgets" how to swim. Later he can slowly relearn how to relax and enjoy swimming. Similarly, women are taught to fear childbirth and have to be trained to relax during labor in order to enjoy the experience.

PAIN IS A PART OF LIFE

Pain is an uncomfortable subject. No one wants it, yet to one degree or another everyone has it.

In our society there is a great emphasis on the complete avoidance of pain ("At the first sign of backache take . . . pills") almost to the point that we forget that pain can be valuable. Pain can be our body's way of telling us that something is wrong and that we need to respond in some way. If you cut yourself shaving, you feel pain, see blood, and respond by applying pressure to the wound to soothe the pain and stop the bleeding. If you sprain your ankle you have pain that increases greatly when you try to walk on it. You respond by not walking until the ankle has healed enough to tolerate your weight.

Your response to pain is affected by the intensity of the pain. The greater the intensity, the more likely you are to do something to stop it. But how you view that pain also affects your response. The marathon runner who finishes the race experiences pain, and knows in advance that he will, but this does not stop him from running. The pride and sense of accomplishment he has is worth the discomfort.

Pain has several degrees of intensity, and we encounter them often. First, there is the pain that makes us *uncomfortable*. You trip on the stairs and twist your ankle. It is bothersome, but you can cope with it. The next level of pain is that which *hurts*. You realize that you did not just twist your ankle, but that you badly sprained it. You wrap it, put ice on it, elevate it, and avoid walking on it for a while. It is inconvenient and it hurts, but again you can cope with it. The third degree of pain causes *suffering*. This type of pain may be encountered in a severe auto accident. This is incapacitating pain—a pain we cannot cope with. This is the pain we fear and do our utmost to avoid.

Almost daily we experience a pain that we consider uncomfortable, and sometimes we have pain that actually hurts, but we do not fear these pains. We do not lie in bed afraid to get up simply because we may experience some pain. We know that these pains may affect what we do that day, but we can cope with them. This is the type of pain you will encounter in labor. At first, the contractions will tug a little, and later they may ache or hurt. However, with preparation, the pain will not be unbearable. You will not suffer. You do not have to fear the pain of labor.

One factor that increases the intensity of all pain, little or great, is fear. All of us fear pain when we do not know how much there will be, how long it will last, or what to do about it. This fear of the unknown can be one of the greatest sources of pain in labor. Your Lamaze preparation will provide you with complete knowledge of the anatomy and physiology of childbirth, as well as the progress of labor and birth. By preparing yourself well in advance, you will know what happens during labor, approximately how long labor will last, and best of all, what to do to prevent or avoid pain.

You will carefully practice the Lamaze techniques of breathing, relaxation, concentration, and stroking so that you will be prepared to use them automatically during labor. The purpose of these activities is to allow you to labor more comfortably and efficiently. The more thoroughly you practice, the more confident and relaxed you will be when labor begins, and the more effectively you will use these techniques to cope with your sensations.

You may think, "I can't do that. I'm not that strong a person. I'll chicken out in the end and won't be able to go all the way." There is no such thing as success or failure in childbirth. Please do not make "going Lamaze all the way" your goal. The true objective of preparation is the joyous, safe birth of a healthy baby. Every labor is different. If your labor is such that the techniques you have learned do not carry you through, you will not be a failure if you enlist the aid of medication. Remember your goal, and do not allow the expectations of others to interfere. You want a satisfying experience—one that you can remember with joy. If you go into labor convinced that you will not use medication, you may feel like a failure if your labor is such that you require some assistance during it. You cannot predict what the experience of labor will be. An informed, open mind will allow you to use whatever is necessary to obtain the best possible birth experience.

The perfect medication for use in labor—one that has no adverse effect on the baby and allows the mother to fully experience the birth without discomfort or side effects—has not yet been found. All medications have the potential to affect the baby in some way. Medications that enter the mother's bloodstream also enter the baby's system through the placenta. This is true for those drugs that the mother takes by mouth (PO), by injection into her muscle (IM), or by intravenous drip (IV). If the effect on the mother is to relax muscles or make her tranquil or sleepy, the same effect occurs in the baby to some degree. The closer to birth these medications are given, the longer they may remain in the baby's system; his system is immature and will take time to eliminate them.

Another factor to remember is that individuals react differently to these medications. A small dose may assist one mother in relaxing and enable her to continue her techniques more effectively, whereas the same dose may make another woman drowsy and decrease her ability to control her sensations and reactions.

Medications do play a useful role in labor when there is a need for them. It is difficult to decide whether to take or refuse medication during labor. Ideally, you should discuss the subject with your birth attendant prior to labor. Once he knows what your goals are, he will be in a better position to help you achieve them. You and your birth attendant are members of the same team working toward the same goal. Before requesting medication, assess your progress. You may be further into labor than you think! If you are doing well and do not feel that you need medication, you will not be forced to take any. The safest, most effective analgesic is the loving encouragement and guidance of your partner and birth attendant.

A WORD TO FATHERS

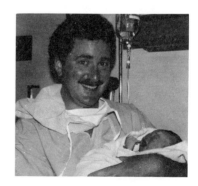

Why should you become a member of this team? For many years, fathers were restricted to the waiting room for most of labor and all of birth. Today, many men feel dissatisfied with this. They want to be with their wives. Others, however, think that having a baby is "women's work." They feel that they have finished their jobs, and, furthermore, they can't stand to see their wives in pain. Besides, the sight of blood makes them sick.

First of all, your work has just begun! Being a father is a big responsibility. Sometimes fathers who attended their children's births report that their birth experiences have made fatherhood more satisfying. The child has become not "hers," but "ours."

For someone who has never had a child, it is difficult to imagine what contractions feel like. The apparent intensity of your wife's contractions can be awesome. You may feel helpless when confronted with such an experience. In addition, seeing someone you love in pain can be very frustrating. However, these feelings of helplessness and frustration may not occur if you assist your wife during childbirth. Your wife will be able to cope with or avoid pain if she carries out her techniques, but a woman in labor cannot always think clearly. Your wife may need your help to interpret the progress of labor and react appropriately. Furthermore, your emotional support may be crucial if she is to get the maximum benefit from her techniques. To read more about what you can do to make your wife more comfortable during childbirth, see pages 114–117.

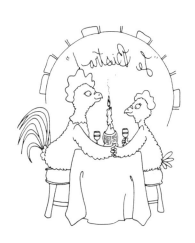

You and your wife may have many misconceptions about labor and birth. During labor there is no "blood and gore"—only contractions. During the birth there is some blood—your baby will have a slightly bloody fluid on his head as a result of small blood vessels in the cervix that break during his passage down the birth canal. In your classes, you will see pictures of birth and will understand what we mean. At the time of your own child's birth, however, you will probably not even notice any blood. Both you and your wife will be very busy. You will be at her side, encouraging her, appreciating her efforts, and sharing the joy of your baby's entry into the world.

In addition to the benefit of a more comfortable labor, Lamaze preparation for childbirth may even enhance the relationship between husband and wife. Statistics cannot measure the effect of this type of childbirth on the marital relationship. However, many Lamaze couples state that they have "fallen in love" again.

THE HISTORY OF CHILDBIRTH PREPARATION

Lamaze is a method of childbirth preparation involving education, techniques, and support designed to make childbirth a more comfortable and rewarding experience. Labor and birth can only be comfortable if pain is decreased or eliminated. Lamaze preparation attempts to eliminate some of the causes of discomfort, thereby eliminating some of the pain.

For many centuries, pain was thought to be a *necessary element* of the birth process. Not until the 1800s did anyone analyze women's labors in an effort to determine the validity of this assumption. Only then did they realize that pain was not an essential part of labor. Attempts were then made to relieve labor pains. Hypnosis was used first, with varying degrees of success. Later, medications were used with the same mixed results.

In 1920, an English obstetrician, Dr. Grantly Dick-Read, attended a young woman who appeared not to have any pain during her labor and delivery. He was impressed, and when he questioned her, she replied, "It wasn't meant to hurt, was it?" Her comment haunted him each time he attended a woman who labored in agony. Why had the young woman experienced no pain? Slowly, he came to believe that childbirth was not supposed to involve suffering. Women have a uterus for the sole purpose of conceiving and bearing children. If the uterus performs as designed, why should there be suffering, anymore than when the lungs breathe, the heart beats, or the intestines digest? If there is pain during digestion or breathing, then there is something wrong with the organ. The abnormality could not be in the design, but must be caused by some outside factor. Dr. Dick-Read theorized that the problem lay in the mother's reaction to labor—she was afraid, and consequently tensed her muscles when she experienced contractions. He felt that this tension deprived the uterus of the oxygen needed for nourishment, causing the uterus to starve. He concluded that pain could be eliminated during labor if the woman relaxed, and that she could relax if she were not afraid. Dr. Dick-Read educated his patients and taught them how to relax and breathe. His approach worked for some. However, because fear is not the only cause of pain in labor, not all women were helped. The term "natural childbirth" was used by Dr. Dick-Read, who is considered to be the father of prepared childbirth.

About the same time that Dr. Dick-Read was preparing his patients for labor in England, experiments with dogs and conditioned reflexes were being performed in Russia. The experiments were to have great significance for childbirth preparation as we know it today. Dr. Ivan Pavlov found that dogs could be made to respond in a predictable fashion to a specific stimulus if the stimulus was combined with the same response often enough. A dog salivates when food is placed in his mouth. This is an unconditioned reflex, one that the dog was born with. But the type of food for which he salivates is learned. Puppies raised on milk alone do not salivate when given meat until they learn that meat is food also. Then the sight, smell, and taste of meat make them salivate. This is a learned or conditioned reflex.

A more complicated learned reflex is salivating at the sound of a bell, but this is easily accomplished if the dog is fed every time a bell is rung. Soon he learns that "bell equals food." A new pathway of stimulus-response has been formed in his brain.

Humans, too, become conditioned to respond to specific stimuli. Because we are smarter than dogs, we do not have to physically experience everything. We can learn by just hearing words. If a child burns his hand once, he learns what "hot" means. Later you need only tell him that the pan, match, water, or fire is hot, and he will avoid them.

You wonder what drooling dogs, bells, and burned hands have to do with childbirth? A great deal! These all involve learned or conditioned responses. You will respond to the contractions of labor with certain learned or conditioned responses. For instance, during your classes, you will be conditioned to think "muscle contraction," not "pain."

In 1945, Russian physicians began employing conditioning with almost all of their obstetric patients. A French obstetrician, Dr. Fernand Lamaze, visited Russia and observed the effectiveness of this approach to labor. In 1952, he imported the techniques to France. He made some changes, and the news of his techniques spread throughout the world. His approach became known in the United States in 1955 when Marjorie Karmel wrote her book, *Thank You, Dr. Lamaze.*

The technical name for this technique is the Psychoprophylactic Method of Preparation for Childbirth: Psycho = mind, prophylactic = prevention. This is a method of preventing pain in labor by conditioning the mind or brain.

DEALING WITH PAIN IN LABOR: THE LAMAZE TECHNIQUES

The causes of pain in labor fall into two categories: emotional and physical. One emotional cause of pain is prior conditioning. We have already learned from the words of others how to deliver our babies. We do it with much suffering! This prior conditioning is one of the primary causes of pain during labor.

Both men and women think "labor pains" when they think of labor, because that is what contractions are commonly called. There is not one of us who does not respond with some fear when we think of some pain we are about to endure. Think of how you respond when you prepare to go to the dentist. (Our apologies to dentists everywhere who do not produce pain. Many of us still worry.) We avoid making appointments, are conveniently late, or "forget" about going altogether. Women worry about childbirth, too, but cannot forget about going into labor.

Women often go into labor expecting pain and fearing its intensity. This fear produces the undesirable cycle of fear-apprehension-tension-muscle spasm-pain-fear of greater pain, and so forth.

We have been conditioned to respond to fear with tension. We prepare to either fight or run from that which frightens us. But there is no way to fight or run from the uterine contractions of labor. Muscles that remain tense become painful. If you hold your arm out with all muscles firmly contracted for several minutes, you will find that your muscles ache. Many unprepared women feel aches all over after birth because of tension during labor. The unprepared woman feels panic when she has a contraction that hurts. She holds her breath and her body automatically tenses. When the contraction ends, she should relax; but, because she is not sure when the next onslaught will be, she remains tense. She may relax just as the next contraction begins, thus being caught unprepared. Eventually she does not relax at all. Fear affects the brain adversely, causing pain to be experienced with greater intensity.

Another cause of pain that is closely associated with fear is the mother's reaction to the sensation of uterine contractions. Women are often amazed by the strength of contractions and become fearful because they did not anticipate it. At full term, the uterus is one of the largest muscles in the body. This organ has grown from two to three ounces to two and a quarter pounds. When most muscles contract they move a joint, but the uterine muscle works differently. The contractions pull at the cervix (or opening of the uterus) to thin and stretch it until it is large enough to allow the baby's head to emerge. The sensations from the uterus will be different from any you have previously experienced. The contractions of labor are very strong. If they were not, the cervix would not open and your baby would not be born.

The uterus contracts throughout pregnancy. At first, the contractions are not noticeable. These early contractions help the uterus to enlarge with the growing baby. Later they prepare the uterine muscle for labor. You will become more aware of these contractions (called Braxton-Hicks contractions) as you get closer to your due date.

The contractions of early labor are often like these non-labor contractions. Many women go to the doctor for their scheduled appointment experiencing mild sensations, and then go directly from there to the hospital because they are in labor. Suddenly the contractions become "labor pains." They are not different from those experienced before, but now the labor is influenced by the mother's reaction to the fact that she is in the hospital and by the lack of control she has over what is happening to her. Many women associate hospitals with pain and illness. It is important to remember that there are no such things as "labor pains." There are only uterine contractions. They may be painful, but they are still contractions. If you think "contractions," you may have some contractions that are not painful and some that are. But if you think "pain," you will be more likely to have painful contractions only.

These emotional causes of pain in labor will be somewhat eliminated by the knowledge of what can be expected during the various stages of labor. You will know that there are some things that you can do to control what happens to you during your childbirth, and you will get a chance to tour your birthing area so that you will be familiar with it, and thus far less apprehensive about your hospital stay.

Some of the physical causes of pain can be eliminated also. One of these is the interference by the surrounding muscles of the abdomen and diaphragm with the activity of the uterine muscle. The contracting uterus swells, just as the biceps in your arms swell when they contract. But unlike the biceps, which are covered only by skin, the uterus is covered with strong abdominal muscles. Muscle groups tend to copy each other. When the uterus contracts, the surrounding muscles reflexively contract and provide resistance to the uterine contraction. To prevent this you will practice controlled relaxation exercises, which will enable you to release the abdominal muscles during labor. You will also perform a light stroking of the abdomen, called effleurage, which helps relieve tension in these muscles.

Because the diaphragm, which lies beneath the lungs, is necessary for respiration, you cannot relax that muscle. Each time you inhale, the diaphragm goes down. As you exhale, the muscle comes back up. The superficial chest breathing you will use during labor is very light and rapid, and will keep the movement of the diaphragm to a minimum while providing the maximum amount of air exchange. This will relieve pressure on the uterus from above.

Another physical cause of pain in labor is an insufficient oxygen flow to the uterus. Every muscle uses oxygen to burn glucose, which in turn produces energy. If there is not enough oxygen, the glucose is not completely utilized, and converts to lactic acid. A build-up of lactic acid results in muscle swelling which, in turn, causes pain through pressure on the nerve endings. If you ever went on a crash exercise program, you may have experienced this sensation. You probably exercised excessively the first day, and when you finished were terribly winded but felt good because you were sure that you would soon see the results. You did. The following day, you were so sore you could hardly move.

The same thing can happen to the uterine muscle during labor. If the uterus does not get enough oxygen, the muscle becomes irritable and pain occurs with each contraction, especially as labor progresses and the contractions become stronger. But this pain is unnecessary and can be avoided by supplying the uterus with adequate oxygen. All athletes learn how to increase their breathing as they exercise. In labor, you will increase your breathing rate as the uterine muscle works harder and the contractions grow stronger.

As labor progresses, the baby will be pushed down into the pelvis, producing rectal or pelvic pressure and, perhaps, an urge to push. This urge may occur before the cervix has dilated (opened) enough for the baby to emerge. Pushing at this time would press the baby's head against the softer ring of muscle, the cervix. This can produce pain. Although the urge to push may seem overwhelming, you can overcome this urge by repeatedly exhaling, quickly and forcefully. You will automatically inhale after each exhalation. This pattern will prevent premature pushing and the pain that may accompany it.

In addition to altering your breathing, you must relax your entire body during contractions. Every muscle that works needs oxygen. Unprepared women attempt to fight their labor contractions. Tension then interferes with the contractions and causes pain. No matter how hard you fight, your uterus will continue to contract. The only satisfactory alternative is to relax. But you must practice relaxation in advance of labor. You have no control over the activity of the **smooth muscles**, e.g., those of the uterus and intestines (much as you might like to tell the uterus to stop and give you a rest). However, you can control the **striated muscles**—those which are attached to the arms, legs, face, neck, and other body parts. These are the muscles you will learn to control during labor so that they remain relaxed.

During birth, as your baby moves farther down, pressing upon and stretching the vaginal opening, a strong stretching sensation will occur. Your reaction may be to tense the pelvic floor, or perineum, to prevent tearing. This tension may cause a tear in the vaginal opening, which will surely cause pain. If your pelvic floor remains relaxed, however, the pressure of the baby's head will cut off the blood supply to the nerves in the area, causing the area to numb. Through practice, you will be able to relax your pelvic floor for the delivery.

Your baby's position in the uterus may be another cause of pain during labor. If your baby is lying with his back toward your back (in a posterior position), you may experience a severe backache during contractions. Your baby may lie this way not because he is being perverse, but because this position enables him to fit best into the uterus or pelvis. Because he has to rotate so that his back is toward your front for birth, labors involving this position are usually longer and more uncomfortable. There are several things you can do to relieve this backache and assist the baby's rotation. These are discussed on pages 90–94.

There may be other causes of pain in labor not yet identified. To overcome these, you will maintain a high level of activity in the cortex of your brain. The brain accepts only so much stimulation and then ignores or eliminates new signals. The most complicated signals take priority.

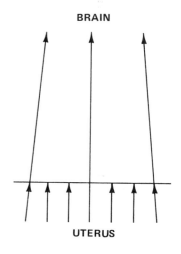

BRAIN

UTERUS

Figure 1.1
Barrier to Sensation.
Breathing, relaxation, and concentration techniques prevent the brain from perceiving most pain impulses.

The beginning of a contraction will be your signal to start breathing, relaxing, concentrating, and stroking before the contraction reaches its peak. These techniques will take priority and will close the gate to other stimuli, namely the uterine contraction. To understand this phenomenon, think of a time when you had a headache before watching a good movie—or before getting involved in some other enjoyable activity—and then forgot about your discomfort during the movie, only to find after the movie that the headache had not really disappeared. The movie had temporarily taken priority, causing the headache to be ignored. The Lamaze breathing and relaxation techniques are difficult to perform, and therefore are capable of creating a level of activity sufficiently high to prevent most pain impulses from being acknowledged. You will know that you are having a contraction, but will not feel its full intensity.

We have outlined the reasons for performing certain techniques during labor, but you are probably still wondering how and when they should be done. Before we pursue these points, you might find it helpful to understand the anatomy and physiology of the uterus, and the basic mechanics of the birth process.

Chapter Two
Pregnancy

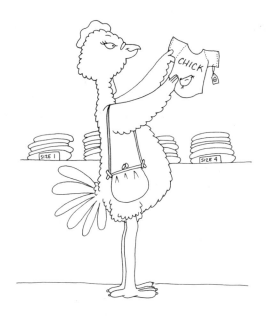

Pregnancy is a forty-week journey for both you and your baby. As your baby grows from a cluster of cells to an active fetus, so does your own body change, both internally and externally. Increasing your knowledge about your body and your baby's growth can increase your confidence, and that confidence can make both the preparation for birth and the birth itself easier.

Although your body was designed to give birth, this process is not without its discomforts. Usually, exercise and good nutrition can alleviate the minor discomforts of pregnancy. Exercise tones your muscles for pregnancy, prepares you for birth, and aids in your postpartum recovery. Beginning an exercise program now, during pregnancy, may establish a lifelong habit for you, your partner, and your baby.

This chapter first discusses the anatomy and physiology of pregnancy. It then explains the prepared childbirth techniques that can help to make your pregnancy and birth more comfortable.

MATERNAL ANATOMY

As you look at the illustration of the baby in the uterus on page 15, you should note several things. Greatest in size is the baby, who is lying with his head at the bottom of the uterus and his buttocks at the top. This is called a **vertex position**. Most babies assume this position about the eighth month of pregnancy, probably because the head is heavy and sinks. They usually stay this way until they are born. If the baby is lying in the uterus with his buttocks at the bottom and his head up, he is in a **breech position**. About three percent of all babies assume and maintain this position. The next thing you should notice is the dark outline around the baby. This is the **uterus**. Before pregnancy, the uterus weighs about two ounces. During the pregnancy the uterus not only stretches to accommodate the growing baby, but also grows, so that at full term the uterus is one of the largest muscles in your body, weighing about two pounds. This growth is due to the formation of new cells, the enlargement of already existing cells, and an increase in the blood supply to the uterus. Is it any wonder that you are more aware of the uterus contracting during labor than you are of your thigh muscles contracting when you walk?

The uterus itself is composed of three groups of muscles: the longitudinal (up and down) muscles, the oblique (diagonal) muscles, and the circular muscles. Functions of the uterus include cradling the baby inside the mother during pregnancy, protecting him from injury, and pushing him into the world during childbirth.

The **cervix**, or the opening into the uterus, protrudes into the **vagina**, which has an external opening. In front of the uterus is the bladder, and behind the uterus is the rectum. Although you cannot see it in the picture, the opening into the uterus at the cervix is closed with a plug of mucus. This **mucous plug** prevents germs and other foreign matter from getting into the uterus and keeps the environment sterile for the baby. The plug may be released shortly before or during labor.

The next structure to look at is the **placenta**. The placenta, which allows for the exchange of nutrients and fetal waste, is composed of many blood vessels. There is no mixing of the mother's and baby's blood through these vessels.

The placenta looks like a flat disk, and is about one half to three quarters of an inch thick and about seven to nine inches in diameter. The flat surface that is attached to the wall of the uterus looks much like liver. The other side of the placenta, which faces the baby, has the amniotic sac attached to its surface. It is smooth and shiny, and resembles liver that has been covered with gray cellophane. Large blood vessels spread over this surface after branching out from the umbilical cord.

The **umbilical cord** is attached to the placenta, usually in the center. The cord is about two feet long and is composed of three blood vessels: two arteries, and one vein. It is covered with a substance called **Wharton's Jelly**, which feels like very stiff gelatin. When exposed to air, this jelly expands and clamps off the blood vessels within. The blood vessels are longer than the cord

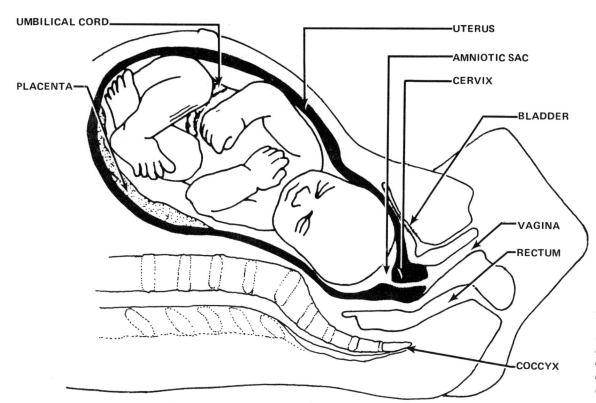

UMBILICAL CORD

PLACENTA

UTERUS

AMNIOTIC SAC

CERVIX

BLADDER

VAGINA

RECTUM

COCCYX

Figure 2.1
The Baby, Prior to Labor
Before labor, the cervix is long, hard, and thick. No effacement or dilation has taken place. The baby's head is not yet engaged in the pelvis.

itself, and on examination you can see them spiraled throughout the length of the cord. This prevents tension on the cord from placing tension on the blood vessels.

The placenta and umbilical cord form the life-support system of the baby until he is born. The baby's waste products are eliminated via the umbilical cord and placenta. Through this system he also receives all his nourishment—oxygen; sugar, vitamins, minerals, amino acids, and fatty acids from the foods his mother eats and digests for him; and antibodies, which fight disease. He also receives substances that are harmful to him through this system, such as nicotine from cigarettes, caffeine, drugs, and alcohol. At one time, the placenta was considered to be a barrier to all toxic elements. Today we know that almost anything that gets into the mother's blood stream also enters the baby's blood via the placenta and umbilical cord. This is why there is so much concern about drinking, smoking, and drug use during pregnancy.

The baby lies in a sac of fluid called the **amniotic sac**, or **bag of waters**, throughout the pregnancy. This fluid provides an environment of constant pressure and temperature for the developing infant. It also protects the baby in the event of a blow to the mother's abdomen by spreading the pressure throughout the uterus. (Have you ever tried hitting someone under water in a swimming pool?) Even though he may kick back to let the mother know that the insult was not appreciated, blows do not usually cause injury. The baby also drinks and urinates into this fluid. This fluid is continuously absorbed and replaced by the placenta.

Although we call this the amniotic sac, it is really composed of two membranes, the amnion and chorion, separated by a thin layer of fluid. The sac is very resistant to blunt pressure, so your baby can't kick a hole in the sac. Once an opening is made during labor, the amniotic sac tears easily. Thus, the sac does not hinder the baby's progress out of the uterus.

The uterus is supported in the abdominal area by three sets of ligaments. The **broad ligaments** extend from either side of the uterus to the hipbones. The **round ligaments** extend from the front sides of the uterus and end in the groin area. The **uterosacral ligaments** extend from the back of the uterus to the sacrum, the lower flat part of your spinal column that is below the waistline. These do not hold the uterus rigidly in place, but they do support it.

As you study Figures 2.2, 2.3, and 2.4, note how the bladder and rectum are affected as the baby moves downward during childbirth. Both become very compressed so that there is little room in either organ. During labor you must remember to urinate frequently, because there will not be enough room to store much urine. A full bladder could obstruct your baby's descent or make the contractions feel stronger than they really are. Many women hesitate to push forcefully during birth because they fear the embarrassment of having a bowel movement at that time. Relax. As you can see, very little fecal material can get past the blockage produced by the baby's head. (See Figure 2.4 on page 19.) Additionally, many women experience a natural cleansing of the lower bowel through diarrhea in early labor, while others may be given an enema. The result is that there is frequently no fecal matter in the bowel to be expelled during the pushing phase.

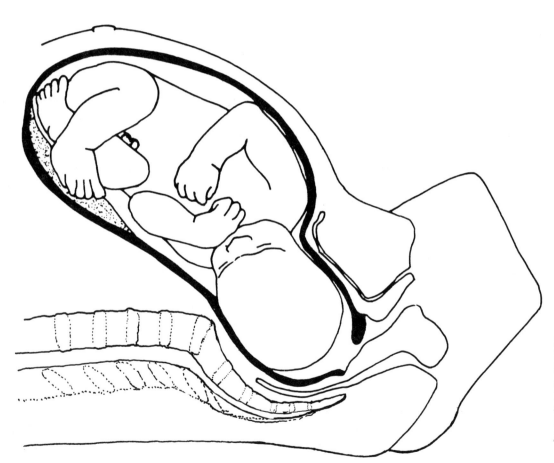

Figure 2.2
The Beginning of Labor
Effacement is almost complete and the cervix has dilated about 3 cm. The baby's head is now engaged and in position to begin its passage through the pelvic bones.

Another structure of significance during the birth is the **coccyx**, the last segment of the spinal column. This small bone is attached to the sacrum with cartilage that cushions the two bones. The placenta produces a hormone that causes this cartilage to soften and become more elastic, thus allowing the coccyx to be pressed downward as the baby moves down the birth canal. You can see this by comparing Figure 2.1 on page 15 with Figure 2.4 on page 19.

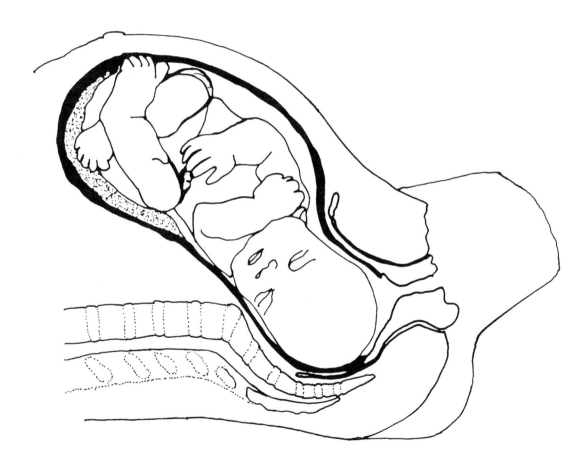

Figure 2.3
The Middle of the
First Stage of Labor
Effacement is complete and the cervix has dilated to about 7 cm. The baby is descending farther into the pelvis.

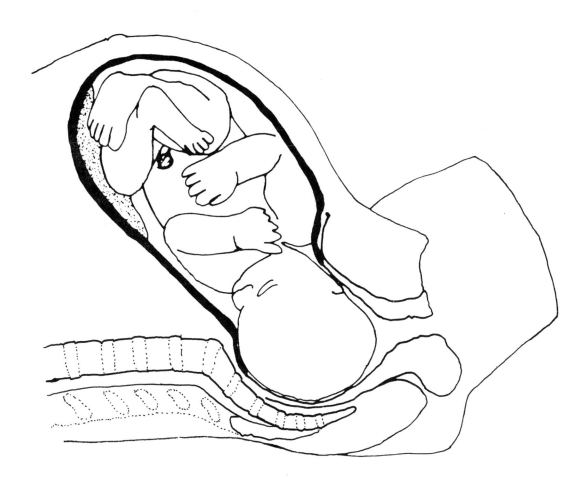

Figure 2.4
The Second Stage of Labor
Delivery—the second stage of labor—has begun. The cervix is completely dilated and the baby has begun his journey down the birth canal.

Figure 2.5
The Pelvic Floor
Comprised of a group of ham-
mock-like muscles, the pelvic
floor supports the reproductive
organs.

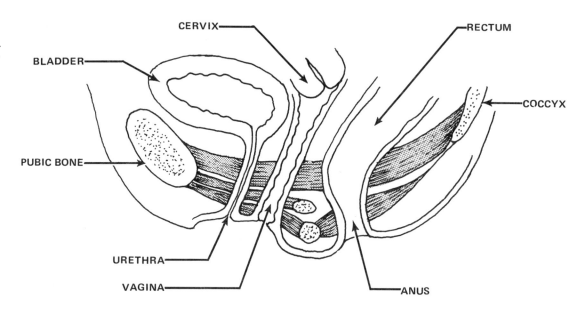

The **pelvic floor** (see Figure 2.5, above) is comprised of a group of muscles that support the bladder, uterus, and rectum. Visually similar to a hammock, it is attached to the pubic bone in the front and the coccyx in back. There are three openings in the pelvic floor: the urethra, which goes from the bladder to the outside; the vagina; and the anus. When you want to stop urination or bowel movements, you contract the pelvic floor.

The **bony pelvis** is composed of the innominate bones (the hipbones), the sacrum (a triangular bone comprised of five fused vertebrae), and the coccyx. Cartilage cushions the area in which the coccyx joins the sacrum, as well as the area in which the ilium (the uppermost portion of the hip) and sacrum are joined (the sacro-iliac joint). There is also cartilage at the junction of the right and left hipbones, in the front. This is the symphysis pubis, or pubic bone.

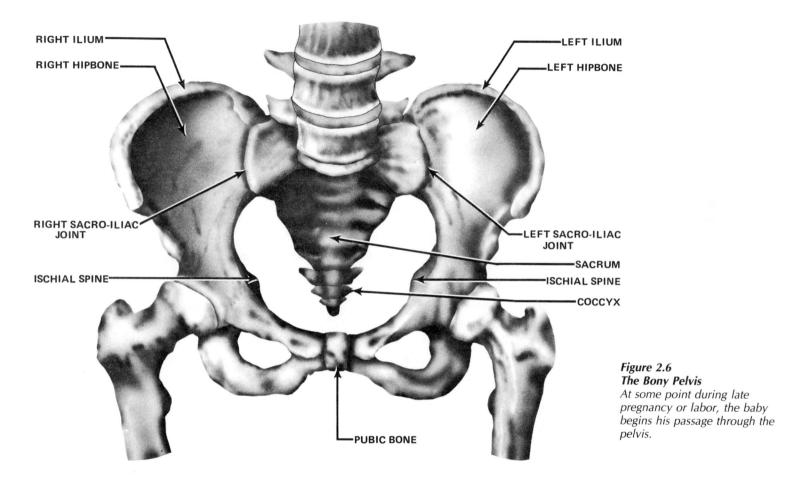

RIGHT ILIUM

RIGHT HIPBONE

RIGHT SACRO-ILIAC JOINT

ISCHIAL SPINE

LEFT ILIUM

LEFT HIPBONE

LEFT SACRO-ILIAC JOINT

SACRUM

ISCHIAL SPINE

COCCYX

PUBIC BONE

Figure 2.6
The Bony Pelvis
At some point during late pregnancy or labor, the baby begins his passage through the pelvis.

The **ischial spines** are bony knuckle-like protrusions on the inner right and inner left sides of the pelvis, at about the level of the cervix. They cause the pelvis to be narrow from side to side at that point, and wide from front to back. These ischial spines are the markers by which the baby's descent is measured.

FETAL ANATOMY

I will praise thee.
For I am fearfully and wonderfully made . . . Psalm 139:14

Before we get very far into this text, we should explore what is happening to your baby now, and what occurred before.

Conception and the First Trimester

Neither blaring trumpets nor fireworks announced the beginning of your baby's life. Most likely, you were sleeping, satisfied and content in each other's arms, your lovemaking complete, sleeping the sleep of the just-after. But under this surface calm, much activity was going on in the mother's body.

During orgasm, the father-to-be sends millions of tiny sperm into the vagina of the mother-to-be. These tiny sperm furiously race around, trying to swim upstream to the egg. With a life span of about 48 hours, they have to hurry. Swimming about three inches per hour, the sperm first travel through the cervix, then up the uterus to the fallopian tubes located on each side of the top of the uterus, and finally up the fallopian tubes to the expectant egg—a distance of about eight inches. Most of the sperm do not complete the journey. Many get lost in the uterus or take the wrong turn and end up in the wrong fallopian tube. But one sperm makes it.

The egg has been recently released from the ovary as part of the menstrual cycle. This little egg (really about 90,000 times larger than the sperm, and just barely visible to the naked eye) has not really been waiting, but has been slowly making her way down to the uterus. She has a life span of 12 to 24 hours, and probably is not too excited until all those sperm appear! What a lucky gal! Since she has only 23 chromosomes of the 46 necessary to grow into an embryo, she needs the 23 chromosomes provided by the sperm. Once the sperm and egg combine, they are a complete unit. After about 24 to 48 hours, they split into two cells, and thus begins the wonderful transformation from egg and sperm to your beautiful baby.

Your baby's first couple weeks are not easy though. They are fraught with danger, the most serious being that the mother's body may reject the developing embryo, not realizing what he will mean to her nine months later. Initially, the fertilized egg moves down the fallopian tube, increasing the number of cells as he goes, but staying the same size as the egg. When the morula, a raspberry-like cluster of cells, reaches the uterus about three to four days later, he quickly burrows into the lush lining that has been prepared for him and covers himself over with it. He has to hurry. The lining is due to detach and produce the menstrual flow in about ten days. But since he intends to stay, he has to stop that. So, he sends out a signal—a hormone HCG (human chorionic gonadotropin)—to the mother's body to tell her to make another hormone (progesterone), which will prevent the uterus from contracting and pushing him out. He then sends out villi to tap into the nourishing lining of his mother's uterus for his oxygen and nutrients. (After all, that is what it is there for. Each month during menstruation the old lining is shed and a brand new one begins to form, so that it will be ready to sustain a new life.) These finger-like villi also help anchor the morula firmly in place in the uterus.

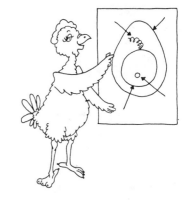

At 15 days of age he has completed **nidation**, or implantation, the process of attaching himself under the uterine lining. Blood vessels are forming and he has stopped your menstruation. In a couple of days, you may begin to suspect that something has happened. Some of you greet this with great and unbounded joy, and others with fear. But your baby, now called an **embryo**, is totally unaware of your reaction to his presence. He is still very busy developing. He has about 266 days to produce about 200 million cells.

At the end of 3 weeks, the embryo looks like a tube with three layers. The outside layer, called the **ectoderm**, will form the skin, hair, sweat and oil glands, and nervous system. The middle layer, called the **mesoderm**, will produce muscles, bones, blood and lymph vessels, kidneys, sex organs, and blood. The third inner layer, called the **endoderm**, will develop into the digestive tract, urinary system, and lungs.

Your baby is very tiny—only 6 millimeters, or about 1/10 inch in length—by the end of the fourth week, but already his heart is beating. It really begins twitching at about 18 to 21 days, and is now pumping his blood around. His heart is very large because it has to pump through the placenta as well as the baby's little body. His head is large in relation to the rest of his body—about one-third the entire length. Lung buds and the gastrointestinal tract and spinal column appear. The eyes, circulatory system, thyroid, liver, and kidneys have begun to form.

If he could, the baby would warn his mother about the dangers of alcohol, drugs, and tobacco to his rapidly developing body. But, of course, he cannot talk. At this point he does not know anything either. He has insufficient brain growth for that.

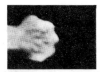

Hand plate—5 weeks.

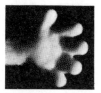

Finger ridges—6 weeks.

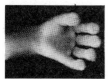

Definite thumb and fingers with pads—7 weeks.

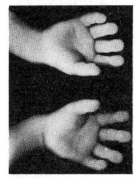

Regression of finger pads— 12 weeks.

Figure 2.7
The Development of Baby's Hands

You may not know about these dangers either. Women of childbearing years should take good care of their bodies, avoiding excessive use of drugs, alcohol, tobacco, and radiation, and maintaining good nutrition. You should always be prepared, because you never know when you may conceive. Once you are aware of conception it is advisable to avoid exposure to all hazardous substances.

While your baby has only one to two cells that will eventually become an organ, the danger of damage to that future organ is great. Later, if one to two cells are damaged it will not have the same consequences, because the thousands of other cells can compensate. Although many women have taken drugs during the first three months of a pregnancy with no resulting problems, we do not know the drugs' long-term effects. It is therefore wise not to take *any* drugs, unless they have been prescribed by a physician who knows you are pregnant. Recent research indicates that alcohol is dangerous for the developing baby even when taken in small amounts. Smoking mothers may have smaller babies than mothers who do not smoke. You may think, "Oh good, I want a little baby. I'll smoke." But if his small size is due to a lack of oxygen in his blood, what other systems are also affected? For your own peace of mind as well as for your health and that of your baby, it is best to avoid these toxins.

At 5 weeks, your baby begins to reveal human characteristics as the ears, jaw, nose, and eyes take shape on his face. His arms and legs are now paddle-shaped buds. The umbilical cord begins to form, and the placenta begins to function. The baby's brain is growing rapidly, and cranial and spinal nerves are developing. Because of this rapid brain growth, you must make sure that you eat well. "You are what you eat" is one saying that has great significance for your baby. The more protein, vitamins, and minerals you eat, the more you make available to him. Pregnancy is *not* the time to go on a diet. When you diet, your unborn baby diets too, but his needs for good nourishment are paramount now.

Many things happen during the sixth week of your baby's life. He is only slightly longer than 1 centimeter (cm)*, or ½ inch, and weighs about ¹⁄₃₀ ounce. His eyes are open. He has a tiny mouth with lips, a palate (the roof of the mouth), and buds for 20 teeth. His nostrils have formed. His fingers have reached the first joint, but are still webbed. His feet are not as well developed.

*2.54 centimeters = 1 inch.

The reproductive organs of ovaries and testes are there, and the penis is beginning to form on the little boys. The ribs start developing from the spinal column forward. All the internal organs of the adult are present in various stages of development. A top layer of skin is forming over the beginning muscles. Nerve impulses for reflex actions (like the knee jerk) are being established. All this has happened, and you have only just missed your second period!

At 7 weeks, bone cells begin to replace the cartilage in the jaw, ribs, and vertebrae, and your baby starts to move his muscles in a coordinated fashion. Up until now, his blood cells formed in a yolk sac, but now the liver has developed sufficiently to produce new blood cells, and the yolk sac has degenerated.

At 8 weeks, the process of organ formation (organogenesis) is complete, and bone is rapidly replacing cartilage in the baby's body. For these reasons he is no longer considered to be an embryo, but is called a **fetus**. Of course, you always think of him as a baby, but technically others do not.

At 8 weeks, the fetus is about 3 cm in length (slightly longer than 1 inch), and weighs 2 grams (1/10 ounce). His eyes are closed, and will remain so until the seventh month to protect them as they finish developing. Unlike the kitten who can't see at birth because his eyes are still closed, your baby can see.

The baby's arms and legs are well developed, but tiny. Each arm is just long enough to touch his face, but not his other arm. He moves around a great deal, but because he is so small you cannot feel it yet. If you could see the baby now you would know whether to choose a girl's or a boy's name, as the genitalia are now recognizable. His heart has four chambers and beats 40 to 80 times a minute.

Between the eighth and twelfth weeks of his life, your baby's muscle and nerve coordination improves, making his movements smoother. He now inhales and exhales using his rib muscles, but cannot drown because he does not depend on air in his lungs. He receives all his nutrients—including his oxygen—from his mother's blood, through the placenta and umbilical cord. His kidneys work to make urine, his pancreas makes insulin, and his liver secretes bile. His liver, spleen, and bone marrow make all his blood cells. Fingernails and toenails begin to grow, and his arms and legs are approaching their final form.

At the end of the first trimester (the first 3 months of pregnancy), your baby is about 9 cm (3½ inches) long from head to rump, and weighs about 40 grams (1½ ounces).

Foot plate—6 weeks.

Toe ridges—2 days later.

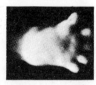

Heel development—7 weeks.

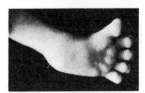

Appearance of walking pads—8 weeks.

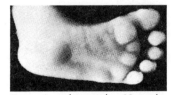

Regression of toe pads—12 weeks.

Figure 2.8
The Development of Baby's Feet

The Second Trimester

During the second trimester (13 to 26 weeks) your baby continues to develop rapidly. During the fourth month (13 to 16 weeks) the musculo-skeletal system matures greatly, and since the baby is bigger and more active, you may begin to feel movement. Your baby's fingerprints and footprints have developed. The baby's heartbeat can be heard with a Doptone amplified stethoscope. He sucks his thumb and swallows amniotic fluid. He weighs between 160 and 200 grams (5½ to 7 ounces), and is about 14 cm (6⅓ inches) long.

During the fifth month (17 to 20 weeks) your baby develops hair on his head, as well as eyebrows and eyelashes. His whole body is covered by *lanugo*, a fine downy hair, most of which will be rubbed off before birth. The oil and sweat glands in his skin function to produce *vernix*, which is a cheese-like coating that will protect his delicate skin while he floats in water for 4 more months.

At this time he also develops a sleep/awake rhythm, which frequently is the same as yours. He may also have a favorite position to lie in. Because of his size, which has more than doubled since the fourth month, you may be able to distinguish a foot or arm pressing against your ribs. The baby may go through crying motions, but since there is no air to move through his larynx, he makes no noise. By 20 weeks he weighs about 460 to 500 grams (about 1 pound) and is 19 cm (8½ inches) long.

During the sixth month (21 to 24 weeks) of your pregnancy, the most dominant occurrence is the significantly increasing formation of bone in your baby's skeletal system. Make sure that you provide adequate calcium for bone growth and development. Good sources of calcium are milk, cheese, yogurt, dark green vegetables, nuts, sardines, oysters, and clams.

At this time the baby also develops certain reflex reactions, such as the startle reflex, which makes him react to loud noises, and the grasp reflex.

At the end of the sixth month the baby weighs from 650 to 820 grams (1¼ to 1¾ pounds) and is 23 cm (10½ inches) long.

During the seventh month (25 to 28 weeks) the eyes completely develop and the eyelids open and close over them. There is not much to see inside the uterus—just darkness. The lanugo is being slowly rubbed off. The testes begin to descend into the scrotum.

By the end of the twenty-eighth week, your baby weighs about 1,000 to 1,200 grams (2¼ to 2½ pounds) and is 28 cm (10½ inches) long.

The Third Trimester

During the last trimester (29 to 40 weeks) several things happen. The baby grows from about 13 to 20 inches in length, and triples his weight. There is great subcutaneous (under-the-skin) fat production to insulate him and help keep his body temperature regulated outside the uterus.

During the eighth month he gains about ½ a pound per week. He stores great quantities of iron for blood formation after birth. With this in mind, make sure you have adequate iron and calories in your diet for his needs.

The central nervous system and brain develop greatly now. The lungs mature by producing alveoli, the structures in which oxygen and carbon dioxide are exchanged. The gastrointestinal system matures.

During the ninth month, an increased amount of maternal antibodies to diseases such as measles, mumps, rubella, whooping cough, and scarlet fever are sent though the placenta to the baby. These antibodies will protect him throughout the first 6 months of his life. You may not have had these diseases yourself as a child, but may have received vaccinations to give you an immunity to them.

You may wish to use these last months of your pregnancy to identify different aspects of your baby's personality. He probably has the same sleep/awake pattern that you have. When he is awake, what does he do? Is he active or quiet? What kind of things seem to irritate him? Does inactivity bother him? Does he start kicking after you have been sitting quietly for a while, or after you have been standing still? Does he tell you that it is late and that he wants to go to sleep? After you have been moving around a great deal, does he tell you that he wants you to take it easy for a while? What kinds of activities seem to soothe him? Does he like the motion of walking or rocking in a chair? Does he like being massaged or sung to? You may find that many of the things that soothe him now will do so after he is born.

Your baby is very busy during the 9 months of pregnancy. He develops from a single fertilized egg, produced by 1 egg and 1 sperm, into a 7½-pound, 21-inch long package of joy! The old cliché about good things coming in small packages still holds true. Your baby will be small, but his power to affect your life and body will be great. Let us now explore some of the ways he affects your body and life during the pregnancy.

PHYSICAL CHANGES DURING PREGNANCY

Many changes occur in your body during pregnancy. The most obvious one is the increasing size of the uterus as the baby grows. As a result of this enlargement, the blood vessels in the pelvic region may be compressed, thus producing varicose veins; edema, or swelling, in the legs; and leg cramps. The intestines are pushed beside and behind the uterus, which may produce constipation. The stomach may be forced upward, producing shortness of breath and heartburn. Frequency of urination may result from pressure on the bladder.

The heavy uterus changes the mother's center of balance, and she adjusts her posture and gait by leaning backwards to avoid toppling forwards. This may result in back and shoulder aches. In addition, the enlarged uterus sometimes strains the ligaments that give it support, producing pain in the back (from the stretching of the uterosacral ligaments) or groin (from the stretching of the round ligaments). The uterus may also place stress on the lower abdominal muscles.

Lung capacity increases during pregnancy as the rib cage expands. The breasts also increase in size as the body prepares for nursing. The breasts usually become smaller after birth or nursing, but the rib cage may not.

Many women find that their fingers and feet become larger during pregnancy. This may be partially due to swelling. During pregnancy, the body retains extra fluid and the volume of blood increases to accommodate the increased need for nutrients of mother and baby. After birth this swelling goes away. Even so, some women notice that their hands and feet remain slightly larger than they were before the pregnancy.

The placenta produces hormones that are geared to maintain the pregnancy. One of these is progesterone, a smooth muscle relaxant. This hormone is produced primarily to relax the smooth muscle of the uterus, thereby preventing it from contracting and dislodging the baby before he is ready for birth. Because the bladder, intestines, and stomach are also composed of smooth muscle, they too are affected by this hormone. As a result, some women experience constipation, a need to urinate frequently (possibly due to an incomplete emptying of the bladder as well as decreased capacity), and heartburn. Heartburn is caused by the slowed emptying of the stomach.

The placental hormones also cause softening of the cartilage in the pelvis so that the pelvis becomes more flexible, allowing more room for the baby's passage during birth. A disadvantage of this greater flexibility is that pressure may be exerted on the sciatic nerve, causing pain and weakness or numbness along its path from the center of the buttocks down through the legs.

With all these physical changes occurring, it is no wonder that many pregnant women are uncomfortable, especially during the last couple of months of pregnancy. What follows is a description of the more frequent physical complaints and some suggestions for relief.

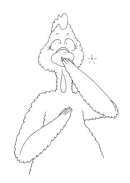

Heartburn may be experienced after meals, particularly if you lie down. You can avoid the burning sensation by eating smaller, more frequent meals; drinking less fluid with your meals; and remaining upright for one hour after eating. Avoid foods that are spicy, greasy, carbonated, or high in sugar. Do not take baking soda for relief because of its excessive sodium content. Any milk product may help to relieve heartburn. A tablespoon of yogurt is especially effective. Your doctor may prescribe a suitable antacid if you need one.

Shortness of breath may be relieved by raising your arms above your head and breathing with your chest muscles. Good posture, with your chest held forward and shoulders back, will help. At night you may be most comfortable sleeping with several pillows under your head.

Frequent urination is common in both early and late pregnancy. One reason for these frequent nighttime visits to the bathroom is that while you sleep the circulation from your legs improves, sending more blood through the kidneys and producing more urine. To prevent bladder infection, urinate whenever you feel the urge. Make sure that you completely empty the bladder.

Varicose veins, which are enlarged, swollen veins, may be visible, or you may simply feel aching and fullness in your legs. Walking often on your tiptoes may help your circulation and reduce this problem. Maternity support hose can be very helpful, especially if you put them on before getting out of bed in the morning.

Hemorrhoids are varicose veins that develop in the rectum. Plenty of exercise—especially walking—and a good diet (adequate amounts of fluids, fresh fruits, coarse fiber-rich vegetables, and whole grain breads and cereals) may prevent constipation, which can aggravate hemorrhoids. If you are plagued with hemorrhoids, lie with your buttocks elevated on a pillow for 10 to 20 minutes, several times a day, and do the pelvic floor exercise described on page 34.

Edema, or swelling, may be prevented by eating a good diet, avoiding excessive amounts of salt on your food, and elevating your legs for 10 to 20 minutes, several times a day. It is unnecessary to restrict fluid intake.

Leg cramps may be easily relieved by straightening your knee and pulling your toes toward your head, thus stretching the cramped muscle.

Dizziness may occur while lying on your back because of the pressure of the uterus against the aorta and inferior vena cava. If this occurs, change your position. Also, avoid getting up too quickly from a sitting or reclining position.

Varicose veins, edema, leg cramps, and **dizziness** may be relieved by wearing loose clothing, lying with your legs elevated at a 45 degree angle, or lying on your *left* side as often as possible. The **inferior vena cava,** the major blood vessel carrying blood from your legs to your heart, lies on the right side of your body near your spine. Lying on the left side allows the weight of the baby to be supported by the bed and eliminates pressure on this blood vessel. To lie on your left side, extend your left leg, keeping your knee straight, with your right leg flexed 90 degrees and elevated on a pillow. Your left arm should be behind your back, if possible. This position also relieves that heavy, aching feeling sometimes experienced in the abdominal muscles. You may lie on your back if both legs are flexed and supported by pillows. If you are working and cannot lie down, sit with your legs elevated whenever possible. A foot massage will also help the circulation in your legs.

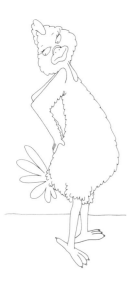

Backache can be prevented or relieved by maintaining good posture. Wear flat or low-heeled shoes and stand tall with your abdomen pulled in. Because poor abdominal muscle tone contributes to backache, use the exercises for increasing abdominal muscle tone (pelvic rock and bent leg raises) presented on pages 34 and 35 to make yourself more comfortable.

Using your body properly when getting up or lifting objects may also help prevent backache. When getting up from a reclining position, avoid doing a sit-up, which can strain the abdominal and back muscles. Instead, take a deep breath, hold it, roll over to one side without twisting at the waist, and get up on your hands and knees; now breathe out. Straighten your back, and stand up. Squat, do not stoop, when picking up objects and children from the floor. When you squat, your back is straight and your legs do all the work. If you forget and stoop, then remember that you are not supposed to do that, drop one knee to the floor, straighten your back, and stand, using your leg muscles. If you are picking something up, bring the object as close to your body as possible before rising from the squatting position. Tailor sitting on the floor, with your legs crossed in front and your back rounded, will decrease the exaggerated curve in the small of your back and relieve tension in these muscles. If you already have a backache, the pelvic rock and Shiatsu, or thumb-pressure massage, described in the next paragraph will help you greatly.

Thumb-pressure massage (a form of Japanese acupressure called Shiatsu) is a type of back massage. It may be more effective than the conventional way of giving a back rub, and you may find that it enables your entire body to relax.

Sit tailor-style with your elbows resting on your knees for support and your body completely relaxed, or lie on your left side with your lower leg and arm straight behind you and pillows under your head and flexed upper leg. Your partner should then place his thumbs at your neck and feel for the grooves on either side of your backbone. The area in which you will be massaged extends from the neck to approximately four to five inches below the waist.

With the flats of his thumbs, your partner should press firmly into the grooves. His thumbs should not slide up or down or rub in a circle, but should press *straight in*. This firm pressure should be held for a count of three. Then, moving down one thumb-width at a time, your partner should proceed slowly to cover every inch of the spinal grooves. He should press with his thumbs only; the other fingers must be held away from your back. Do not push back against your partner's thumbs, but stay relaxed. Pressure should be firm, but not to the point of producing pain. If it hurts, the amount of pressure should be reduced slightly until you feel no discomfort. The massage should move down your back about three times during each session.

Both men and women will benefit from this form of massage. Try it when you have a backache, nervous tension, or trouble sleeping. You will be amazed by how good you feel afterwards. Shiatsu can also be very soothing in labor when used to relieve backache and tension.

Sciatic pain, or pain in your buttocks that travels down your leg, can be relieved by doing a pelvic twist. Straddle a chair, facing its back. Put your left arm across the back of the chair in front of you, and extend your right arm behind you, holding the chair near your left buttock. Keep your head in line with your body as you slowly and gently twist to the right; then return to the starting position. Repeat this several times. Change arms and twist to the left. This will realign the pelvic bones. Do this exercise several times a day to relieve your discomfort. Proper posture will also help prevent sciatic pain.

Severe cramping in the groin caused by muscle spasms in the round ligaments may be noticed when you are walking or when you stand up quickly. It may cause you to bend over in pain, thus relieving the cramp. If you can, sit down and lean forward, or lie down with your legs elevated. You need to decrease the distance between the uterus and the groin to relieve the spasm. You may not be able to sit or lie down if you are shopping for groceries or whatever. In that case, lean forward, raise one knee, and step on the cart, or just squat down and pretend to get something from the lowest shelf. Pregnant women do have their difficult moments!

Neck and shoulder strain may also be a problem. Again, this may be due to poor posture, so straighten up! In addition, you can do the "windmill" or "angel" exercise to relieve this tension. Stand with your back touching the wall and your feet flat together on the floor. Begin with your arms at your sides. Slowly slide your hands against the wall and over your head as you inhale, and slide them back down as you exhale. Repeat several times. You may also do this while lying on the floor. This exercise is not for pregnant women only, but will benefit anyone with back or neck tension.

Occasional sleeplessness plagues many pregnant women. This may be due to the baby's activity, a limited number of comfortable sleep positions, heartburn, shortness of breath, frequent awakenings to go to the bathroom, worry, etc. Avoid taking over-the-counter medication. Instead, try a warm cup of milk or herbal tea, a brisk walk followed by a warm bath, or a dull book. You may also try Shiatsu or a back or foot massage to relieve tension and encourage relaxation.

The previous discussion focused on the most common discomforts of pregnancy. If you have any others, your birth attendant may have some suggestions for relief. These techniques are not meant as a substitute for good prenatal care. You should inform your birth attendant of these discomforts at your regular checkup. If you experience sudden and severe swelling, a persistent headache, or vision disturbances such as blurring or dimming, you should report these immediately. Other symptoms that should be immediately reported are severe abdominal pain or cramping, vaginal bleeding, and the absence of fetal movement for 24 hours. These occurrences are not common, and may indicate an underlying problem that needs treatment.

The following exercises, too, may relieve many of your discomforts while preparing your body for labor.

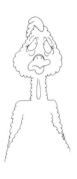

EXERCISES

Rest is important during pregnancy, but many women go overboard in their attitude toward rest and completely eliminate exercise from their lives. By the time they go into labor, their bodies are ready to retire, with muscles that are weak and flabby. Physically, they are certainly not ready for labor! Labor is hard work, and should be prepared for as you would prepare for any other type of hard work. Remember, you are going to be in "the ocean" for several hours. You will soon study how to swim, but you may not be able to paddle—or even tread water—unless your muscles are in shape.

The following exercises are designed to improve the tone of those muscles needed for labor and birth. They will also relieve some of the discomforts that occur so often during pregnancy, particularly toward the end, and insure a more rapid figure recovery after birth. Any exercises that you perform should make you feel better after you do them. These exercises will increase the circulation throughout your body and provide a good exchange of air in your lungs. You will feel refreshed and alive again.

Practice daily! Wear loose clothing, and either wait at least one hour after eating to exercise or exercise before meals. Start off gradually and increase daily until you reach the suggested number of repetitions. Some of these activities should be done as often as possible from the very beginning of pregnancy.

Pelvic Elevator (Kegel)

This is an extremely important and effective exercise. Its purpose is to develop elasticity and muscle tone of the pelvic floor and to heighten your awareness of tension and relaxation. If the pelvic floor muscles (see illustration on page 20) are slack, the bladder may slip backward into the vagina as the uterus drops downward and the rectum slides forward. By exercising this muscle group you will provide proper support for your pelvic organs, and they will stay in place.

Perhaps more important to you now is that exercising the pelvic floor will provide a more comfortable pregnancy by increasing the circulation in your groin and alleviating pelvic congestion, which, if left untreated, can result in varicosities of the vulva (the area around the vaginal opening) and rectum. Birth will be more comfortable because you will develop a greater awareness of tension in and relaxation of the pelvic floor muscles, and thus will be better able to consciously relax them. Contrary to what you might expect, the more tone a muscle has, the more thoroughly it can relax. This will be very important to you as you push your baby out during birth. A well-toned pelvic floor stretches more easily, resulting in a smaller episiotomy, or no episiotomy at all. Also, doing the pelvic floor exercises right after your baby's birth will increase circulation to the area, and thus may decrease swelling and speed healing.

Set up a schedule of when this exercise should be done. For example, decide that you will do it every time you open the refrigerator, each time you go to the bathroom, whenever you answer the phone, and so forth. This exercise may be done in any position: sitting, standing, or lying down. Practice it at least ten times a day, beginning today. With increased muscle tone and awareness, intercourse also may be more pleasurable, especially if you practice while making love.

Pretend that your pelvic floor is an elevator that stops at every floor of a busy building. To allow the elevator to go up, slowly but steadily tighten the pelvic floor as though preventing yourself from urinating and defecating. This will not involve the muscles of the abdomen, back, or legs. Take a deep breath in and out. Then breathe normally: first floor (pelvic floor relaxed) . . . second floor (contract your pelvic floor slightly) . . . third floor (tighter) . . . fourth . . . fifth (lots of people getting on—hold it) . . . sixth floor (pelvic floor as tight as you can make it) . . . fifth (release muscle slightly) . . . fourth . . . third . . . second (almost there) . . . first floor (totally relaxed) . . . basement (push out) . . . quickly up to third floor (slightly tense). Take a deep breath. Wasn't that fun?

The second part of this exercise is the "express elevator," which starts on the first floor, goes directly to the sixth floor and stops for a while to let a large group of people on, and then goes directly to the basement to let them all off. Quickly return to the third floor to wait for the next group. Begin and end with a deep breath. Become an express elevator at least 50 times each and every day for the rest of your life.

Pelvic Rock

This is a valuable exercise for anyone who has a backache from work or tension. It also increases the muscle tone of the abdomen—which will help you to push during birth—and may relieve some of the lower abdominal heaviness that is frequently felt toward the end of the pregnancy. You may also find this exercise helpful in labor if you experience a backache during contractions.

Lie on the floor with knees drawn up and feet flat on the floor. Use no pillows. Take a deep breath in, and exhale. Breathe in again, and as you slowly blow the air out, pull in your abdominal muscles and flatten your back against the floor, keeping your legs relaxed. Your labor partner can check your position by placing a hand under the small of your back. When the exercise is done properly, you will be pressing hard against his hand. Hold your back down for a slow count of five; then release your back and abdomen as you inhale. Repeat as you breathe out. Do this ten times, ending with a deep breath in and out.

You may do this exercise as often as you want for the relief of backache. Once you understand the basic pelvic movement, you will be able to do this on all fours, standing, or sitting.

Tailor Press

The tailor press exercise will help prevent your thighs from aching after the birth. This will be especially important if stirrups are used to support your legs during birth. The tailor press stretches the ligaments of the thighs, increases circulation to your legs, and improves muscle tone. The abdominal muscles, also, will benefit from this exercise.

Take off your shoes and sit tailor-style on the floor, with the soles of your feet together in a comfortable position. Place your hands under your knees, palms up. Take a deep breath in and out; then breathe normally. Slowly press your knees toward the floor as your hands push upward against your knees. Hold for a count of five; then gradually release your knees to the starting position. Repeat five times, ending with a deep breath. Begin gradually and work up to ten repetitions a day.

Over and Out (Bent Leg Raising)

This exercise is good for everything. Abdominal and leg muscle tone is increased, backache is relieved, and circulation in your legs is improved, decreasing fatigue and swelling.

Lie on the floor with your knees bent and feet flat. Do not use pillows. Take a deep breath in and out. Now breathe in again. As you breathe out through pursed lips, raise one knee over your abdomen—"over and out." Feel the pelvis rock? Maintain the pelvic rock as you breathe in and raise your leg, straightening the knee and pointing the toes towards your head. As you exhale, contract your abdominal muscles to keep your back from arching, and flex your foot as you lower your leg to the floor, keeping the knee straight. As you breathe in, slide your foot to the starting position. Repeat with the other leg; then relax your pelvic rock. Begin gradually, increasing to ten times a day with each leg.

PREPARING FOR CHILDBIRTH

You are now aware of basic female anatomy and the process of pregnancy, of some of the discomforts of pregnancy and the exercises that may be done to relieve them, and of what can be done during the pregnancy to help assure a healthy mother and baby. Now we will discuss how to prepare for a happy childbirth experience. We will begin with a brief explanation of the process of labor, followed by in-depth coverage of the techniques you will use, the reasons for their use, and the way they should be used during labor.

The Process of Labor

Labor is a fairly simple process. Figure 2.1 on page 15 shows the baby lying upside down in the uterus—the most common pre-labor position. The baby does not fall out, because the bottom of the uterus (the cervix) has a very narrow opening that must be greatly enlarged to allow him to pass through. The primary purpose of the labor contractions is to open the cervix sufficiently to allow the baby to leave the uterus.

The first phase of the labor process is the effacement phase. **Effacement** is the thinning of the cervix. Before labor begins, the cervix is about the length of your thumb from the tip to the first knuckle, and about one and a half inches in diameter. In the first phase, the cervix thins to about one eighth of an inch (see Figure 2.2. on page 17). Imagine pulling a tight turtleneck sweater over your head. At first the neck is long and thick. As you pull the sweater down, the neck thins and opens, allowing your head to come through. This same process occurs in the cervix, which has to shorten and thin before it can dilate, or open, wide enough for the baby's head. The shortening and thinning process of effacement continues throughout most of the labor. If this is not your first baby, the cervix may efface and dilate simultaneously.

The second phase of labor is called **dilation**. During this phase the opening in the cervix enlarges sufficiently for the baby to pass through (see Figure 2.3 on page 18). Contractions start at the fundus (the top of the uterus) and travel down to the cervix, causing the cervix to shorten and open. When muscles contract, muscle cells become small. When muscles stop contracting, the cells usually return to their previous size. However, the uterus during labor is different, because when the contraction ends, the individual cells remain slightly smaller than they were at the beginning of the contraction. Through this process of contraction and retraction, each muscle cell in the uterus becomes progressively smaller. These more compact muscle fibers can contract better (practice makes perfect), causing the last phase of the labor, **transition**, to progress more rapidly. During the transition phase the contractions continue to dilate the cervix, but also start to push the baby deeper into the pelvis. The increased strength of these contractions pushes the baby hard against the bag of waters, causing it to break, if it has not already broken. When the cervix has fully opened and the bag of waters has broken, the baby is able to move down the birth canal.

The baby's descent from the uterus through the cervix and down the vagina (birth canal) can be measured during a vaginal examination. His descent, or **station**, is determined by the location of the presenting part (usually the baby's head) in relation to the ischial spines. If his head is level with these spines, he is at a zero station; above is a minus station; and below is called a plus station. At the zero station, **engagement** occurs. At this point, the baby's head can be felt just at the tip of the middle finger during a vaginal exam. This is the approximate level of the ischial spines. This engagement ("dropping") may occur up to two weeks before labor for a first-time mother (a **primigravida**), and either before or during labor for a woman who has had a child before (a **multipara**). Stations are measured in centimeters. For example, a +1 station means that the baby's presenting part is 1 cm past the ischial spines, and thus 1 cm closer to birth. A +4 station means that the baby's presenting part is visible outside of your body, or is "**crowning**."

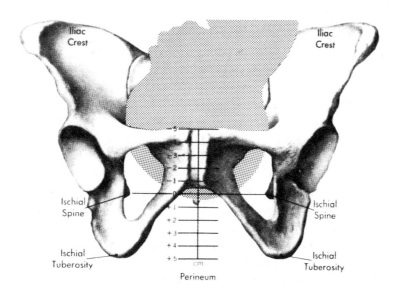

Figure 2.9
Stations of Presenting Part
As the baby descends, his progress is determined by the relation of the presenting part to the ischial spines.

The hormones that are produced during pregnancy cause the muscles of the vagina and pelvic floor to become very elastic. These areas, therefore, open up easily as the baby's head descends. When his head reaches the vaginal opening (the pelvic floor or perineum), the opening dilates, and the baby's head, shoulders, and body are born.

The process of childbirth is not over, however, until the placenta (**afterbirth**) is delivered. After the baby is born, the placenta is no longer needed by mother or baby, so the uterus continues to contract. Because the baby has been born, the uterus now gets very small, causing the place where the placenta is attached to shrink. Therefore the placenta separates and is pushed out. Assistance may be required in the delivery of the placenta. If so, the birth attendant may apply external pressure on the uterus and lift the placenta out manually.

Birth is now complete.

Introduction to Childbirth Techniques

You will be conditioned by frequent practice to respond automatically to your contractions with specific, controlled behavior. Labor is a highly stressful situation, and will demand more effort and hard work than you have ever done before, unless you have had other children. By handling stress effectively, you will conserve a tremendous amount of energy and remain more comfortable throughout labor.

Every skilled athlete practices vigorously before a big event. No sensible person would enter a swimming contest having only read a book on how to swim. Labor is similar. Understanding alone is not enough to enable you to cope with the demands of labor. You must practice to remain afloat. Your body must be conditioned to respond automatically to certain physical and spoken signals, because women in labor may have neither the time nor the desire to think about what the book said. Often labor seems distant and unreal. Some couples make the great mistake of practicing halfheartedly, with grand plans to "hit it hard" later. Remember, your due date is only an estimate. The baby may take you by surprise and come early. So be prepared.

The following techniques are those that you will perform during labor. The more thoroughly you practice them in advance, the more effectively you will employ them in labor. Make a commitment to each other to practice consistently. Working together for this significant event often strengthens your relationship. If you find that Lamaze did not work for someone you know, you should investigate their *commitment.* We can offer the tools, but the real work is up to you.

Relaxation

The ability to relax effectively in labor will assist you in several ways. You must conserve sufficient energy for the effort required to push your baby out into the world. Also, a fatigued body cannot function adequately, as the brain loses the ability to concentrate on the task at hand. There are no coffee or lunch breaks in labor. You go on and on until the job is complete. If you give in to your body's response to "fight" the contractions, you will expend 90 percent of your energy before the job is half done. Concentration and relaxation are the most important as well as the most difficult tasks to continue as labor becomes more intense. However, they form the foundation upon which the other techniques must be built. If, through fatigue, your brain loses the ability to respond, no breathing technique in the world will be of any assistance to you.

Within your body there are two types of muscles. Striated muscles are those that you can control voluntarily, e.g., the muscles of the face, arms, hands, pelvic floor, abdomen, legs, feet, etc. Smooth or involuntary muscles are those that do as they please, regardless of your desires. These include the bladder, bowel, and uterus. As much as you may want to stop the uterine contractions to get some needed rest, you cannot. Whenever a muscle group (voluntary or involuntary) contracts or tightens, other muscle groups instinctively tend to copy the action. When your two-and-a-quarter pound uterus contracts during labor, the rest of your body will tend to tense also. Therefore, relaxation in labor, even though essential, is a completely unnatural thing to do.

During practice sessions, you and your partner will develop an increased awareness of muscle tension and relaxation. You will practice on those muscles over which you do have direct control. Because you cannot tell your uterus what to do, and therefore cannot make it contract during practice sessions, you must pretend that your arms, legs, and other voluntary muscles are your uterus. You can then practice releasing every other voluntary muscle in your body while specific ones are tightened, just as you will relax while your uterus contracts during labor. You will be isolating a group of tense muscles, identifying how far the tension spreads from this muscle group, and learning to recognize this tension so that you can voluntarily eliminate this response and maintain control.

Contracting certain muscles while relaxing all others requires a great deal of practice. In labor, your work will be to mimic a rag doll at the same time that your uterine muscle contracts with increasing force. You will not deliberately contract and relax muscle groups during labor. Your partner will call off these commands only during practice. During labor, he will tell you to relax those muscles that may become tense. Your response to his commands will be automatic in labor only if you rehearse well in advance. Again, women in labor may not have time to reason, so your response to his verbal cues to relax should be so well rehearsed that you can react without thinking. You will begin this relaxation when you feel yourself becoming tense with your labor contractions.

Initially, these relaxation techniques should be practiced while lying on your back on the floor. Place pillows under your head and knees so that all joints are flexed and no strain can be felt in your legs, back, shoulders, or neck muscles. Do not use narrow pillows under your knees, or you will tense up trying to keep your legs from slipping off. (You might also use a reclining chair or chaise lounge.) This is a basic position for practice. After you have achieved proficiency in this position, practice in side-lying and sitting positions.

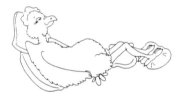

After you are comfortably positioned, select a definite object in the room—a focal point—on which to focus your eyes. Keep your eyes open during these exercises. Focusing on a single object is merely a gimmick to achieve concentration and keep your eyes from roaming around the room and your brain from switching to another train of thought. If you are more comfortable with your eyes closed, then close them, but remember to keep your mind alert. You should concentrate on maintaining tension in those muscles that are supposed to be contracted, and relaxing all other muscles. During labor and practice sessions you should tune in to what is happening within your body and to how you are responding. Begin each practice session with complete relaxation, then move on to active relaxation.

Complete Relaxation

Your partner should kneel closely beside you. He will give you the command "take a cleansing breath" (see page 45 for a complete discussion of the cleansing breath). Breathe deeply in through your nose, purse your lips, and blow out through your mouth. This command will precede and end all relaxation exercises, and the cleansing breath will signal complete body relaxation and readiness to begin. Breathe normally during the actual exercise.

Following the cleansing breath, your partner should check your degree of relaxation. Using the palms and fingertips of both hands, he will stroke the muscles of your body. His hands should conform to the part being touched. Starting with your forehead and face, he will proceed to the neck, shoulders, arms, hands, sides, back, buttocks, abdomen, thighs, calves, ankles, and feet. This stroking should be done slowly, evenly, and rhythmically. He should take a great deal of time stroking each part to really identify the nature of the muscle beneath. Does the muscle feel tight? Loose? Soft? Firm? If you have tension, your partner's job is to help you relax by talking softly and stroking. As he strokes your muscles, let yourself relax under his hand.

To check the neck, your partner should gently move your head from side to side and move his hands over and down the back of the neck. Next, the arms should be checked. After stroking the arm, your partner should firmly grasp your hand or wrist, lift, and shake the arm gently from side to side. If properly relaxed, it will be limp and floppy. He should never drop your arm, as this will cause you to tense and lower it yourself. He should, instead, place your arm on the floor in a comfortable position.

Your partner should next check the legs. There should be no tightness in the knee or hip joints. Your partner should place one hand under the ankle and the other hand under the knee, and slightly lift the knee and gently rock his palm, thus rotating the leg at the hip. He should finish by rotating the foot to insure that the entire leg is relaxed.

Stroking should be done throughout labor. During this exercise, you should concentrate on the stroking and release your muscles to your partner's touch, relaxing each body part as it is stroked. This technique will help your partner to identify any tension in you and will have a very soothing and relaxing effect on both of you. Stroking also provides a physical closeness that will help you to maintain contact with reality. This will become increasingly important as labor intensifies. Many women feel very far away and alone during labor, and the constant touching can help relieve the feeling of being deserted. During labor, the stroking will also produce another set of signals on which the brain can concentrate, and will thus block more of the impulses coming from the uterus during contractions.

Because relaxation is so important during labor, make sure that your partner's stroking is relaxing to you. Tell him whether you want a firmer, lighter, slower, or faster touch, since you cannot relax well if you are being rapidly tickled or slowly steamrollered. This discussion can be just as important as learning how to do the technique itself.

Active Relaxation

After your partner makes sure that you are completely relaxed, he should give you specific commands to contract any muscle group over which you have control. Tighten those muscles as much as possible. Learn to identify tension and relaxation throughout your body, and to consciously relax all muscles that are not supposed to be contracted. Do not relax a group until the command to do so has been given. The command may be verbal, physical (stroking), or both. Because the stroking is a command to relax, your partner should avoid touching the contracted muscle group until he is ready for you to relax it. Your partner will stroke your body continuously, as he did during the practice of the previous relaxation technique. During these exercises you should not talk or smile, as doing so will break your concentration and tighten facial muscles. Wait until he gives you the command for a cleansing breath after the exercise; after the breath, you can speak.

These exercises must be practiced daily with your partner. You will find that practicing alone is also very beneficial. Do this in addition to the sessions together. The more you practice, the better conditioned you will be to relax during labor.

The following is a description of how the different muscle groups should be contracted.

ACTIVE RELAXATION COMMANDS AND RESPONSES

Partner's Command	Mother's Response
• Contract your forehead and face.	• Squint, as though looking at bright sun.
• Contract your neck.	• Push head backwards.
• Contract your shoulders.	• Press shoulders backwards.
• Contract your arms.	• Tighten arms and make fists.
• Contract your hands.	• Let arms rest, but make tight fists.
• Contract your abdomen.	• Pull abdomen in to make yourself look less pregnant.
• Contract your perineum (pelvic floor).	• Pull in rectal/vaginal/urethral openings as if to stop urinating and defecating.

ACTIVE RELAXATION COMMANDS AND RESPONSES

Partner's Command	Mother's Response
• Contract your buttocks.	• Squeeze buttocks together.
• Contract your legs.	• Tighten your leg muscles and bring your toes toward your face. Do not lift your leg off the pillow, as this will tense your back muscles. Do not point your toes, as this may produce a cramp in your calf.
• Contract your feet.	• Spread your toes apart.
• Contract your back.	• Arch or lift your back upwards.

The active relaxation exercise consists of taking a cleansing breath, contracting and relaxing several muscle groups, and ending with a cleansing breath. Repeat the exercise at least four to five times daily.

Breathing Techniques

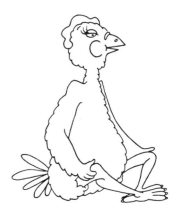

Labor is hard work. During labor, you will adjust the rate of your breathing to the work your body is performing. In early labor, when the contractions are mild, your breathing will be slower than in late labor, when the uterus is working very hard. You will increase your breathing according to how you feel. Since each increase requires more physical and mental effort, stay as long as possible at each level in order to conserve your energy. When you begin having difficulty relaxing and are not getting enough relief, you will know that you should advance to the next technique. This advance is fairly automatic during labor. Remember not to begin your techniques until you can no longer talk through the contractions.

Each technique requires progressively more mental attention, which helps close the gate to impulses coming from the uterus. In early labor, when the contractions are mild and these impulses are few, you will do slow deep, or slow paced, breathing. This is fairly simple, requiring little physical or mental effort. As the contractions get stronger, you will feel that the slow deep breathing is no longer effective and will switch into the second level of breathing, the shallow or modified paced breathing. This breathing requires greater attention and effort. You will move to the third level—the pant-blow or pattern paced breathing—when you find yourself becoming tense and feel that you are not getting enough benefit from the second-level accelerated-decelerated breathing. This pant-blow breathing is mentally and physically the most complicated, and is therefore reserved for the end of labor when you need the greater benefits of this increased concentration.

Always the question arises, "How will I know when to switch?" This is difficult to answer, as there are no guidelines. Some women feel that contractions are strong enough to warrant pant-blow breathing when they have very little cervical dilation. Others do the slow deep breathing until they are almost completely dilated. The intensity of the sensation you feel will determine what breathing you do.

For example, once you learn how to drive a stick shift or manual transmission car, it becomes second nature to you, and you unconsciously know when to shift into a higher or lower gear. If you drive a car with automatic transmission, perhaps thinking of shifting a ten-speed bike will help. In this same way, your body will tell you when to shift breathing levels during labor. Either you or your labor partner may notice that the techniques you are doing are not helping. You may be unable to relax, and begin clutching his arm or the bed. You may become restless and move around because you are not comfortable. Your eyes may roam the room because you are having difficulty concentrating. You may hold your breath or grimace. These are all clues to the need to change your breathing techniques.

The breathing techniques will decrease your perception of the contractions. You will still be aware of the contractions, but will not feel their full intensity. If you doubt that your activity is helping, you can try not using the techniques. Within five seconds you will probably be working very hard to regain control.

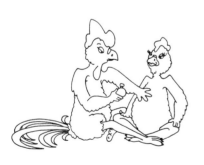

During practice sessions you will simulate contractions. This is done through verbal signals given by your partner. He will talk you through a contraction by calling "the contraction is beginning . . . it is getting stronger . . . it is at a peak . . . the contraction is going away." During real labor, the uterus will provide the signal for your response. Your partner will still tell you when the contraction is beginning, so that you can start your techniques before you actually feel the contraction from within. He can determine the beginning of the contraction by watching the fetal monitor or by using his hand to feel the uterus.

During practice sessions, your partner should also physically simulate contractions. One way he can do this is by giving you a "fire burn." He should place both hands on your lower arm and slowly tighten his grip, twisting his hands in opposite directions (like wringing out a wet cloth), increasing the pressure to a peak, and then gradually releasing the pressure. During this practice contraction you should concentrate on the increasing pressure and on your responses of relaxation, breathing, concentration, and effleurage (see page 47). This is how you will react in labor, adjusting your reactions to the intensity you feel.

Another simulation technique you can try is the thigh pinch. Using his fingers, your partner should slowly and steadily pinch your inner thigh above the knee, gradually releasing it after reaching a peak of intensity. This can be very painful, so take it easy. If you can stand a strong thigh pinch, labor may be a breeze. With these techniques you will learn to respond to physical signals that begin lightly, become more intense, and finally taper off. You do not have to do this with every practice contraction, just occasionally. Your partner should also indicate 15-second time intervals during both practice and labor. A woman in labor loses track of time, and the contractions may seem to last forever. Hearing the time interval helps to set limits on the contractions. This will strengthen your ability to continue until the end of labor.

You should respond to each contraction with total body relaxation, concentration, breathing, and effleurage. Visualize the shape of the contraction as you experience it. This mental picture will help you to respond appropriately and prevent tension. You will know that the contraction tapers off after reaching a peak. Anticipating this decrease will assist you during the peak.

Practice these breathing techniques while lying in your basic practice position. When you feel comfortable this way, practice in the side-lying, sitting, kneeling, and all-fours positions, as well as while standing and walking. Wear comfortable clothes that do not restrict movement. Practicing should not be done on a full stomach; relaxation will not be enhanced.

The Cleansing Breath

Using your chest only, inhale deeply through your nose and exhale through pursed lips, as though you were cooling soup. Allow about five seconds for this breath. If you tried to breathe at one depth for a long time, you would find yourself becoming tense, uncomfortable, and hungry for air. Periodically, you need to take a deep breath to overexpand your lungs. Everyone does this as part of their normal breathing pattern. Did you ever try to pretend you were asleep while someone watched you? Do you remember thinking after a while that you just had to take a deep breath and could not go on with the quiet, even breathing?

This deep breath also helps you to relax. You will take this deep cleansing breath at the beginning and the end of each contraction, because you will not be able to do so during contractions. Your cleansing breath will also mark the boundaries of the contractions. You will relax at the beginning, and if you develop tension during the contraction, your cleansing breath will be the signal to relax again. The cleansing breath is always a sign to relax your body completely, regardless of whatever else you are doing.

Slow Deep Breathing (Slow Paced Breathing)

All the breathing techniques you will employ in labor are done primarily with the diaphragm and chest muscles. The part of the abdomen that is below your navel should not move. Slow deep breathing or slow paced breathing is the first level of breathing, and should be done when the contractions are mild and do not demand much effort to stay above them, but you nevertheless feel the need to use some breathing technique. This breathing is similar to normal breathing. However, it is deeper, slower, and more regular.

Slowly inhale through your nose and blow out through pursed lips. At the announcement "contraction begins," take a deep cleansing breath, relax completely, and fix your eyes on a focal point. Inhale through your nose. Lift your chest up and out. Purse your lips and gently and slowly blow out. Your breathing rate should be six to nine breaths per minute, counting the cleansing breath. The inhalation and exhalation should be even, and there should be no pause in the pattern. When your partner states that "the contraction has gone," take another cleansing breath.

Your diaphragm will move slightly when using this technique, but the interference with the uterus in the early stage of labor will be minimal. Practice for a full minute. Two breaths every 15 seconds is about right.

Effleurage

Effleurage is a gentle stroking of the lower abdomen. It soothes and relaxes abdominal muscles, gives you something to do with your hands, and produces another point of concentration.

Effleurage is done on bare skin. Use powder to help your hands move freely over the skin and to avoid irritation. Stroke the lower abdomen—the area where you are most likely to feel the contractions. Begin above the pubic bone. Lightly stroke with the flats of the fingers up and out toward both hips, then toward the navel and back down to the pubic bone again. In practice sessions, effleurage the area that can be reached when your elbows are resting on the floor (if you are lying down). During labor you will have access to more pillows and will be able to support your arms on them to do the effleurage.

Practice this technique with the slow deep breathing, so that the two automatically go together. Coordinate the effleurage and slow deep breathing as follows: as you inhale, stroke up and out to the hips; as you exhale, stroke to the navel and back down. Begin this technique with your cleansing breath.

This stroking is done throughout labor until transition. Some of you will not want to do this during labor, but will prefer someone else to do it, or will not want it done at all. During transition you will most likely not want to do this yourself, so your partner should assume the responsibility at that time. Whatever works for you is right for you. Practice effleurage anyway, just in case you do want it.

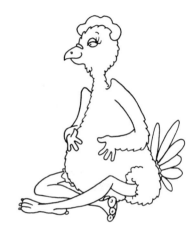

Shallow Breathing (Modified Paced Breathing)

When the slow deep breathing is no longer effective, you will move to the next level, which is shallow breathing or modified paced breathing.

During practice, at your partner's announcement "the contraction is beginning," take a cleansing breath. Push a short breath out at the end of the cleansing breath to further empty the lungs. Do not take a deep breath in, as this will make you tense and uncomfortable during the breathing. Keeping the jaw relaxed and holding your mouth slightly open, breathe in and out through your mouth, up to about four breaths per five seconds (slow rate).

As you breathe, your chest should move slightly. Do not move your lips. You should feel the air just come in and out of your mouth. Do not try to draw it deeply into your lungs. Your breathing should be light, easy, and effortless mouth-centered breathing. The inhalation/exhalation rhythm should be equal. Only the exhalation should be slightly audible. You should not hear your inhalation, but should feel it. Continue for 60 seconds, taking a final cleansing breath when you hear "the contraction is over."

When you feel comfortable with the slow shallow breathing, begin practicing the rapid shallow breathing. This is the same technique as the slow shallow breathing, only faster. Rapid shallow breathing is difficult, and requires a great deal of practice. Practice until you feel comfortable breathing this way for two minutes. The rate should not exceed two to two and a half breaths per second. Again, your partner should signal when the contraction begins and ends. If your mouth gets dry, try putting the tip of your tongue behind your upper front teeth. Add effleurage when you feel comfortable with the breathing. This stroking should be done at the same slow speed throughout. You will be breathing rapidly and stroking slowly, a rather difficult trick to perform at first!

Because contractions first increase and then decrease in intensity, you will modify the speed of your shallow breathing by accelerating and decelerating the rate to follow the character of the contraction (thus the name "modified paced breathing"). This technique will help you to conserve energy, provide you with the proper amount of oxygen at the appropriate time, and serve to increase your level of concentration.

During practice, your partner should time the contractions, signaling their intensity and calling off 15-second intervals. For example, "The contraction is beginning . . . it is getting stronger . . . 15 seconds . . . contraction is at a peak . . . 30 seconds . . . still at the peak . . . 45 seconds, starting to taper off . . . 60 seconds, the contraction has gone." In labor, the uterus will provide the signals for intensity. You should also practice breathing with the "fire burn" or thigh pinch administered during contractions. Begin and end with a cleansing breath. Keep your eyes open, and completely relax your body. As you increase the rate of breathing, you will notice that the breathing becomes lighter and more shallow. When you feel comfortable with this technique, add the effleurage. Remember that the rate of effleurage is independent of your breathing rate.

Figure 2.10 will give you an idea of how your shallow breathing can increase and decrease to keep pace with the intensity of the contraction. During actual labor, your speed will automatically adjust, but you must be careful not to breathe too rapidly or loudly. If your partner notices that you are breathing faster than you did during practice, he should suggest that you slow down. He may help you to slow your breathing by making eye-to-eye contact with you and then

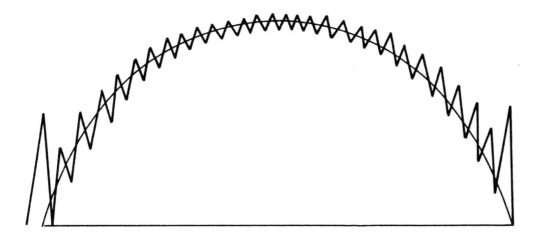

Figure 2.10
Shallow Breathing
You will adjust the speed of your breathing to the intensity of the contraction. As the intensity increases, your breathing should accelerate.

breathing with you, so you can either hear or see him. He may also try tapping out the rhythm on your arm or leg. If this does not help, advance to the next level of breathing for the peaks of the contractions. If you breathe too fast, you will not have time to utilize the air you are inhaling and will hyperventilate and become tense. (See the discussion of hyperventilation on page 74.)

Shallow Breathing Suggestions

1. After the initial cleansing breath, remember to make the first breath an exhalation.
2. Make your breaths short, distinct, quick, shallow, and light, only moving your chest slightly (i.e., keep the breathing mouth-centered).
3. Slightly emphasize each exhalation. This will prevent you from holding your breath, and at the same time allow the chest muscles and diaphragm to relax. Your breathing should be barely audible.

4. It may help to place a slight emphasis on the fourth or sixth exhalation to help establish a pattern.
5. Air intake and output must be equal. Start slowly to get the feel of it. Increase the speed after you have developed a fairly good rhythm and feel comfortable.
6. Watch yourself closely for relaxation. One tense muscle group leads to another.
7. If you start off feeling comfortable, and then feel tense and want to gulp air, you may be holding your breath and contracting your chest muscles. Check your relaxation and slow the breathing rate. You may simply be breathing too fast.
8. If you can't wait to take a deep breath, you may not be inhaling as much as you are exhaling. Blow out quickly three times, slow down, and allow more time to inhale.
9. If you are dizzy, your breathing is too fast and too deep. Slow it down and make it more shallow.
10. Silently count to help keep your breaths equal, e.g., count "one . . . and . . . two . . . and . . . " breathing out on the number and in on the word "and." To speed up the breathing, keep the counting the same but breathe in and out on the number and the word "and."
11. The breathing should be easy and effortless.
12. Be sure to breathe in after each exhalation. Do not force the breath, but let the air flow in.
13. Keep lips and jaw relaxed.

Pant-Blow Breathing (Pattern Paced Breathing)

When labor is at its most intense, you may need to change your breathing to the third level, pant-blow or pattern paced breathing. This technique utilizes the rapid shallow breathing, punctuated intermittently by a forceful exhalation through pursed lips, thereby producing a pattern on which you can concentrate. If you feel the urge to push during this time, you should blow rapidly and repeatedly until the urge has subsided. (Remember that pushing during transition often drains your energy, and may make you uncomfortable.)

Begin practicing transition breathing with six quick breaths followed by a short blow. Be careful not to gulp air in after the cleansing breath or the blow. There should be no pauses or breaks in the rhythm, and inhalations and exhalations should be equal. You will notice that your abdominal muscles tighten during the blowing. This helps relieve the intensity of the feeling that you want to bear down. After blowing out, resume the rapid shallow breathing immediately.

The blowing and counting pattern helps concentration. Practice each contraction for 90 seconds. Your partner should call off 15-second intervals, and should announce "you have the urge to push" twice during the 90-second contraction. After about 15 seconds, he should announce that "the urge to push is gone." This will give you practice with the continuous, repeated blowing. Breathing during transition may involve varying this basic six to one pattern.

As the contraction increases in intensity, you will blow out more often. You may begin your contraction with six breaths to one blow and then change to four breaths per blow, two breaths per blow, and finally one breath per blow, adjusting the pattern to fit your needs. As the contraction decreases in intensity, you will blow out less often. Blow quickly and repeatedly to overcome the urge to push or to keep in control of a very strong contraction. Usually, you will experience the urge to push at the peak of the contraction, when the uterus is contracting most strongly. Practice the continued blowing for up to two minutes so that you can do this in labor, if necessary.

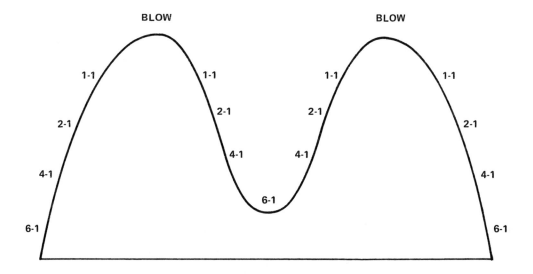

Figure 2.11
Pant-Blow Breathing.
During transition, you will adjust your breathing pattern to the intensity of the contraction. As the intensity increases, you will blow out more often. At the peak of the contraction, repeated blowing will help you to overcome the urge to push.

Figure 2.11 shows how you should breathe during a transition contraction. Start with a cleansing breath, following it with the pattern of six breaths to one blow. As the contraction gets stronger, change to four breaths to one blow, and so on, adjusting your breathing to the intensity of the contraction. At the peak, if you have an urge to push, repeatedly blow out until the urge is gone. End with a cleansing breath.

When practicing pant-blow breathing, your partner should call out the following: "The contraction is beginning . . . getting stronger . . . nearing a peak . . . you have the urge to push . . . the urge is gone, but the contraction is still strong . . . it is tapering off . . . getting less . . . getting stronger again . . . etc." During labor the contractions may vary. To enable you to respond appropriately to any sequence, your partner should vary his commands during practice. You will be better prepared for labor if you experiment with different patterns. Keep your hands relaxed at your sides during practice for transition. Your partner should now practice doing effleurage for you, using one hand to lightly stroke the lower abdomen. No particular stroking pattern is necessary. Your partner should also practice this breathing so that if he needs to breathe with you during labor, he will be comfortable, and not hyperventilate.

Pant-Blow Breathing Suggestions

1. After blowing out through pursed lips, make sure the diaphragm goes slack when you blow out (it will tighten and move slightly), and move the breathing immediately back into your chest. Remember to keep as loose and relaxed as possible.
2. If you find that your entire body is shaking, slow down the breathing and make your breaths less deep. Concentrate on releasing all your muscles.
3. Make the pattern of breathing and blowing smooth, continuous, and rhythmical.
4. Do not inhale a gulp of air after the forceful exhalation. Let your lungs expand effortlessly.
5. Do not involve any movement of the lips in the breathing. Purse them only to blow out.

Pushing Techniques

When the cervix is completely dilated, you will begin to push your baby out of the uterus and down the birth canal. The following material first presents a number of positions that can be used when pushing. It then discusses the actual pushing process.

Positions for Pushing

There are several positions that can be assumed for pushing. Some women squat. This is an effective position, as it allows gravity to help the baby's descent and enables the bones of the pelvis to open somewhat more than they can in other positions. Squatting places little strain on the perineum, helping it to relax as the baby is born. The disadvantage of squatting is that it prevents the birth attendant from easily seeing and assisting the birth.

Another pushing position is the side-lying posture. This is a common position in Europe, but is not often used in the United States. The mother lies on her left side with both knees and hips forward and her right leg supported. This position may be comfortable for the mother, but most birth attendants are not comfortable using it.

Some birthing areas use a birthing chair—a chair that has an opening in the front and center of the seat. The chair can be elevated and tilted back so that the birth attendant can see and assist as necessary. This position is comfortable for the mother and allows gravity to assist in the birth of the baby.

Many women give birth on a delivery table in the lithotomy position. In this position the mother lies on her back with her legs elevated in stirrups. Her head is elevated on one or two pillows. Because it permits the attendant to easily see and assist in the birth, the lithotomy position is helpful when procedures such as forceps delivery are necessary. The disadvantage is that gravity cannot help the baby's descent, forcing the mother to almost push uphill. This position may also place extra strain on the perineum.

Another position for birth that is being used more frequently is a semi-sitting position, in which the legs either are elevated in stirrups or rest on the surface of the bed, with knees bent. This position applies great force downward on the contracting uterus by compressing the abdominal area and pushing the baby out from above. The pelvic floor is also relaxed and thinned.

The Pushing Process

Try to assume as vertical a position as is comfortable for you and your birth attendant (about 45 to 60 degrees), thus allowing gravity to assist your pushing efforts. During practice, lean against your partner or use pillows to support you in a comfortable position. During labor, your partner can elevate the head of the labor room bed. Bend your knees and place them comfortably in front of you. With your hands either under or over your knees, hold your legs apart. To avoid backache and to increase the effectiveness of your pushing, make sure that your lower back and buttocks remain flat on the surface. Keeping your jaws relaxed, round only your neck and shoulders forward while you push. Begin with two cleansing breaths. This will give the contraction time to build to its peak. By timing your pushing efforts to coincide with the peak of the contraction, when the uterus is working hardest, all forces will work together for a faster birth. This technique is called breath-holding.

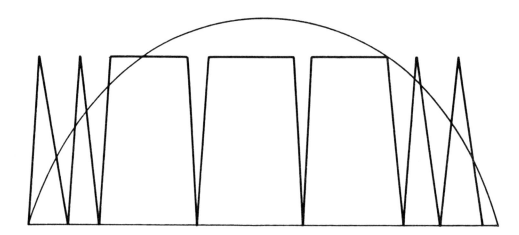

Figure 2.12
Breath-Holding.
During delivery, you will take several deep breaths and hold them while you push. You will probably take 2 or 3 breaths during each contraction.

When your partner states "the contraction is beginning," take two deep breaths. Now take another deep breath in through your mouth. Hold your breath as you round your neck and shoulders forward, and using your abdominal muscles, *push down and out.* Remember to relax your pelvic floor and push through your vagina. Push . . . push . . . push . . . lift your head, let the air out, and take another deep breath. Bend your head forward again and repeat the pushing. During practice sessions, do the actual pushing for a very short time to prevent strain on your body.

When you hold your breath, you will feel considerable pressure in your head. By releasing a little air, this pressure will decrease and the abdominal pressure will increase. This may result in grunting sounds, which many unfortunately consider uncouth. (Oh, that we could be less inhibited about how our bodies work!) Try pushing while releasing some air.

During labor you will push about three times for each contraction, about twenty seconds each time. When the contraction is finished, lie back gently and release your legs. Finish with two or three deep cleansing breaths.

An alternative method of pushing is called gentle pushing. For this, assume essentially the same position recommended for breath-holding, but instead of pushing throughout the contraction, push only when you experience an urge to push. This urge may occur several times during the contraction. If you do not have an urge to push, use the shallow breathing technique.

There are several advantages to the gentle pushing method. The shorter periods of pushing allow for greater blood flow through the placenta than can occur with more sustained and prolonged pushing. The birth is slower, because you only push with the urge to push instead of pushing throughout the whole contraction. This allows more time for the perineum to stretch, often decreasing the need for an episiotomy. But there are a couple of drawbacks. One is that the birth process may be longer and another is that some women do not feel an urge to push at all.

Birth is a very personal experience, and what is most comfortable or effective may differ from woman to woman. Try both of these pushing methods during practice sessions. Then, when giving birth, you will be able to choose the one technique, or the combination of both techniques, that you like best and find most comfortable.

The above pushing methods apply to whatever supine or sitting position you may assume during the birth of your baby. Discuss the available options with your birth attendant. Then, during your practice sessions, try to duplicate the position you will be using for birth. If you will be using a delivery table with stirrups supporting your legs, you might lie on the floor with one to two pillows under your head and your legs resting on a coffee table or the seats of two chairs. There may be handgrips for you to hold onto when pushing on a delivery table, so grab the legs of the chairs and pretend that they are the handgrips.

During the actual birth of your baby, your birth attendant may ask you to stop pushing. This will allow your baby's birth to be more gentle, preventing him from suddenly "popping" into the world. It will also allow more time for the perineum to stretch over your baby's head as he is being born. When you hear the command "stop pushing," you should immediately and gently lie back, quickly exhale, and begin shallow breathing. You will still feel your baby moving down and out of the vagina, because the uterus will continue to push him down, but he will move down the canal more slowly when you don't push.

It is also possible to affect the speed of your baby's birth by altering your position. Due to the effect of gravity, the higher the elevation of your upper body, the faster your baby will move down. The reverse is also true.

After the baby's head is born, the birth attendant may ask you to "give a little push" for the shoulders. To do this, quickly catch your breath, and gently bear down.

Practice this "stop pushing" technique in order to respond correctly while the baby's head and shoulders are being born. If he comes out slowly and gently, there may be less chance of tearing the perineum and less pressure on the baby.

DO'S AND DON'TS FOR PROPER PUSHING

Do:	Don't:
• Keep your perineum relaxed. • Keep your hips and buttocks flat on the surface. (Unless, of course, you are squatting!) • Allow yourself to mentally relax, and let your body give birth.	• Tense your body. • Tense your lips. • Arch your back. • Push without a contraction. • Push as though having a bowel movement. The pressure you feel is only from the baby's head.

The Partner's Role During Practice Sessions

You can get a pretty good idea about what happens during childbirth by reading and attending classes. This theoretical knowledge is nice, but it is not sufficient to get a woman through the strain of labor. Women in labor may not have time to think, and may just react to contractions. Unless the woman thoroughly practices the desired reactions of concentration, relaxation, effleurage, and breathing *before* labor, she may respond to the contractions of labor with tension, either breath-holding or hyperventilation, moaning, and writhing. The decision is yours, but it must be made in advance in order to give you time to practice the techniques. You will get out of it what you put into it!

An athlete planning to enter the iron man triathlon in Hawaii does not prepare by buying suntan lotion, a fancy bicycle, and a bathing suit, but by swimming, running, and cycling. He does not do it alone; he is supported, encouraged, and coached. Sometimes he is pushed very hard by his coach. One man does not win the race by himself. It is a team effort.

Labor is like the iron man competition. In the competition, only one person does the running, but he would fail miserably without his support people. In labor, only one woman has the contractions, but she depends heavily on her support person to inform, coach, provide feedback, and give loving support during the event. This teamwork begins weeks before the event, with daily practice sessions. It takes time and constant repetition.

No matter how tired you both may be, do not skip a day of practice. Your enthusiasm, support, and interest can make all the difference in the world. The teamwork you develop during practice will be essential during actual labor. Use a watch or clock with a second hand when you practice the breathing techniques. Announce "contraction begins" and call out "15 . . . 30 . . . 45 . . . seconds" as well as the strength of the contraction: "it is getting harder . . . it is at a peak . . ." Simulate contractions with the "fire burn" or the thigh pinch. Tolerance will gradually build for the rapid breathing technique. Feelings of discouragement are common initially, but persistence pays off. Think of situations that may occur in labor, such as plateaus, back labor, and induction. Practicing the response to these situations in advance makes it easier to respond to them so in labor. Overemphasize the contraction-relaxation exercises. They may not always seem as hard as the others, and you may tend to go through them quickly. They are *extremely* important, and only with continued repetition will the mother be able to respond to you properly during labor. Make her aware of her level of relaxation, reminding her to relax her facial muscles, neck and back muscles, etc. Command her to contract and then release specific muscle groups. Do the stroking constantly. Remind her to practice the breathing and relaxation in various positions—sitting tailor-style, standing, walking, modified all-fours (see page 91), lying on her back, lying on each side, and sitting in a chair. Not until actual labor will she know which position will be comfortable for her. Practice doing the effleurage for her in case she cannot or does not want to do it herself. Use one hand, moving it in a circular pattern.

As the labor partner, you should be prepared to interpret the progress of labor for the mother.

Read the following section on labor and birth thoroughly. The most difficult time of labor occurs during transition, when the mother's contractions are most intense. If she knows that she is in transition, she should be able to cope better with the contractions. What are the signs of transition? Be prepared to inform her of her progress.

Rehearse what you will do if and when situations arise that appear to threaten the mother's control. Consider how you can respond if she is unable to relax during a contraction. What might you do to help her relax? Try breathing with her, establishing eye-to-eye contact, and having her change her breathing pattern or start blowing. If she does not want to be touched, practice verbally relaxing her. Experiment with different ways of helping her to relax. Discover how you can best make her aware of your loving support. Develop alternative methods of communication, such as speech, touch, and eye contact.

There is little in life more exciting than participating in the birth of a child, especially your own child. However, practicing in advance of this event can be either dull or exciting. It is more likely to be the latter if you "rehearse labor" instead of just "practicing techniques." You can jazz practice sessions up by inventing labor situations and discovering the best responses to them. Plan to use these times together to improve your teamwork and your relationship, as both will be needed for the birth and for the days of parenthood that are ahead.

Chapter Three
Childbirth

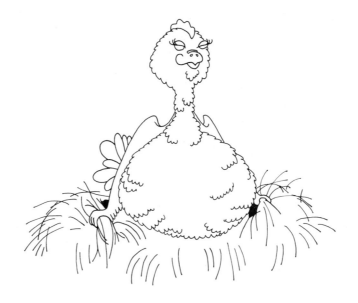

Childbirth is a highly individual experience, as well as a highly emotional one. One woman's childbirth experience—the onset of labor, the length and strength of contractions, the length of labor, the length of time spent pushing, the use of medications and interventions—will not be the same as the next woman's childbirth experience. Childbirth experiences also vary from pregnancy to pregnancy. A long, difficult labor and birth with a first pregnancy does not guarantee a repeat performance with subsequent pregnancies.

What is presented here is the "average" childbirth experience. Of course, the average childbirth experience does not really exist; it is the middle ground of all of the childbirth experiences—the short, the long, the difficult, and the easy. Your experience will not be exactly like the textbook birth described in this chapter. It will, however, have some qualities in common with this average birth. These qualities can help you determine if labor has begun and if it is progressing. A laboring woman is very vulnerable and highly susceptible to suggestion. Your labor partner's sensitivity to this can help him to guide and support you during this time, when the physical sensations of labor can become overwhelming.

LABOR BEGINS

Labor is most likely to begin during the period extending from two weeks before your due date to two weeks after your due date. Your due date is calculated from the first day of your last menstrual cycle. Because you may not remember this date and because some babies are not born 240 days after the beginning of the last period, a due date is not the most reliable indicator of when your baby will be born. Fortunately, there will be signs of impending labor. Naturally, you may not experience all of the possible signs, as each labor is different.

Recognition of Labor

Several things may happen to signal that labor is imminent. They do not mean that you are in active labor—only that you soon will be. When you experience these symptoms, you might get excited, but avoid rushing to the hospital in a panic. You will probably have sufficient time to drive carefully without a police escort.

One of these signals is a **loss of the mucous plug** (called **"show"** or **"bloody show"**). This "show" consists of the thick, jelly-like substance that sealed the cervix during pregnancy to keep bacteria from entering the uterus. As the cervix effaces and begins to dilate, this plug begins to loosen. In spite of being called a plug, it does not pop out like a cork, but rather comes away in small to moderate amounts which you may notice on the tissue after going to the bathroom. This secretion is unlike a vaginal discharge in that it is thicker and may be blood-tinged. Some streaks of blood may be present in the mucus because of the tiny blood vessels in the cervix which break during dilation.

A slight bloody discharge after a vaginal exam late in pregnancy is common, due to irritation of the cervix. If you notice any vaginal bleeding at any other time, however, you should notify your doctor. It may be due to an abnormal placement or early detachment of the placenta. Your doctor will decide the cause and prescribe any treatment needed.

The mucous plug may be lost up to three weeks before labor begins, and be replaced by the mucous-secreting cells in the cervix. Usually, however, it is discharged shortly before the onset of labor or during labor. Loss of the mucous plug without other signals of labor is often insignificant.

The **rupture of the amniotic sac** (bag of waters) is another sign of approaching labor. Depending on the size of the tear in the sac and the position of the baby, you may experience either a gush of fluid or a slow, continuous leak. If you suddenly lose a large amount of water (up to two pints), undoubtedly you will know what has happened. However, a small leak may be difficult to identify. You can distinguish amniotic fluid from urine through several tests. The amniotic fluid is cloudy, has a distinct smell, and cannot be controlled by contracting your pelvic floor. On the other hand, urine is clear, yellow, has a distinct smell of its own, and can usually be controlled. If you are still uncertain, the birth attendant may insert nitrazine test paper into the lower vagina to test the acidity of the vaginal secretions. Vaginal secretions become less acidic when amniotic fluid is present. Do not have intercourse, bathe, or douche if this test is to be done, because the results will then not be accurate.

The bag of waters most often breaks during labor, but may rupture just prior to labor, day or night. If you are concerned about your mattress, cover it with a plastic sheet in case your membranes rupture at night. There is a possibility of uterine infection once the integrity of the bag of waters is broken. Avoid intercourse and check with your doctor about bathing after the bag of waters has broken because of the possibility of introducing bacteria to the uterus and baby. Although a small leak may seal over, usually labor begins shortly after the membranes break. If this does not occur, your doctor may want to stimulate labor artificially.

Because the cushion of water is gone after the amniotic sac ruptures, the baby's head will press more firmly against the cervix. The contractions will then be more intense and more effective. This change in the nature of the contractions is also caused by the fact that the uterus is no longer fully stretched out. You need not worry about a "dry birth," because amniotic fluid is constantly produced until the baby is born.

Before labor begins, some women experience **diarrhea** and **intestinal cramps** and think they have the flu. ("Perfect timing! I'm going to be in labor with the flu!") This may be another sign that labor will begin soon. Diarrhea may be the body's way of emptying the rectum, and the intestinal cramps may be uterine contractions. Because the sensations of intestinal cramping and uterine contractions can be similar, check your uterus to see if it is contracting by placing your hand lightly above the navel. If the uterus hardens at the same time you feel the cramps, you are having uterine contractions.

If you notice a **backache** that comes and goes, place your hand on your abdomen to see if your uterus is contracting. The position of the baby in the uterus may be causing the contractions to be felt only in your back. If you do feel contractions in your back—an occurrence called back labor—refer to pages 90–94 for suggestions about specific techniques to relieve backache.

Because labor usually begins gently and may signal its start in many different ways, it is not surprising that many women have difficulty identifying its onset. True labor, however, rarely goes unrecognized for long. When you experience good labor, you will know that "this is it!" If you have any doubts, then adopt a wait-and-see attitude. You are either in early labor or are having Braxton-Hicks contractions.

Braxton-Hicks contractions occur throughout the pregnancy. Although usually mild and pain-less, they occasionally can be quite uncomfortable. These contractions can be distinguished from true labor in several ways. Braxton-Hicks contractions, which are also called false labor or prelude-to-labor contractions, are usually felt in the abdomen as the skin stretches over the contracting uterus. The contractions of true labor are usually felt deep within the pelvis as the uterus draws the cervix up and open. True labor contractions may initially feel like menstrual cramps, but as they get stronger, they are experienced with greater intensity. True labor contractions may also be felt in the back only, or all through the pelvic area. Other differences between Braxton-Hicks and true labor contractions are the duration of each individual contraction and the total length of time you have contractions. Braxton-Hicks contractions are usually less than 30 seconds in duration; true labor contractions are usually longer than 30 seconds. Braxton-Hicks contractions may come fairly regularly for several hours, but will not become stronger or longer, and will always stop. True labor contractions will not stop until after the placenta is delivered.

Braxton-Hicks contractions often come at irregular intervals, while true labor contractions are usually regular—usually, but not always. If the mother experiences true labor contractions in her back, they may occur at irregular intervals.

Frequently, Braxton-Hicks contractions will change in character or go away completely if you change your activity. If you have been resting, get up and walk; if you have been active, then rest. True labor contractions will not stop.

Contractions that occur at night may feel stronger than they really are, as the absence of distracting activities allows the brain to fully perceive the contractions' intensity. To analyze their true character, get up, drink something, or read a book (perhaps this manual). Do not wake your partner until you are sure you are in labor. He will need his rest in order to be of most help to you in labor. You, too, should rest as much as possible.

True labor occurs when the contractions get progressively longer, stronger, and closer together. All other contractions are probably not labor. The only way to know whether you are in labor is to identify the quality and closeness of your contractions. When in doubt, call your attendant and tell him what you feel.

McKenna's Mystic Rule of Recognition* (the Murphy's Law of labor) states that "If the mother says 'I'm not sure if this is labor,' she is either not in labor or is in very early labor. If, after several false alarms, she says, 'No, this is not labor, I'm sure it isn't!' she definitely is in labor."

Sometimes conditions eliminate the need for you to determine whether or not you are in labor. Your birth attendant may decide to initiate or induce labor and not wait for contractions to begin. One situation that may prompt the attendant to induce labor is the rupture of the amniotic sac without contractions. The closed system that protects the baby is opened by this rupture, and there is a risk of uterine infection if this situation continues. Because uterine infections are difficult to treat, many attendants try to have the baby born within 24 hours of the rupture.

Another reason for induced labor is postmaturity. The placenta has a limited growth potential. After 40 to 42 weeks of pregnancy, its growth may slow. Your baby, however, will continue to grow, and may need more nutrients than the placenta can provide. In this case your baby can thrive better outside the uterus. Other reasons for inducing labor include medical conditions that would compromise the health of the mother or baby if the pregnancy were allowed to continue, e.g., diabetes, Rh sensitization, and toxemia.

What To Do During Early Labor

Once you decide that you are in labor or that you may be in labor, try to rest as much as you can. Being well rested will help you cope later with the physical and emotional stress of labor. If contractions begin at night, try to go back to sleep, or at least to rest. If your contractions begin during the day, you need not jump back into bed, but try not to wear yourself out. Avoid succumbing to the "nesting instinct" that so many women experience before birth. They look at their "filthy" houses and feel compelled to clean them for the mother or mother-in-law who will be visiting after the baby is born. So they begin in the basement and work up to the attic until everything is "spic-and-span." At midnight they flop into bed, exhausted, and begin having contractions at 1 A.M. Labor then becomes an impossible task. Who would be anything but exhausted after all that work? You will waste your energy if you clean before you leave. Get out of your own house and go to a friend's home if you must! You will not respond to this nesting instinct there. Very few women will clean their neighbor's house.

*Mary Jo McKenna, a childbirth educator from Omaha, Nebraska, is credited with the discovery of this law of nature.

If you feel like eating, choose your foods carefully. Select light foods like flavored gelatin, toast, and fruit; and liquids like tea, fruit juice, and soup. During labor, the digestive process slows considerably. Liquids leave the stomach in about one hour, but solid foods take longer. Having food in your stomach may increase the possibility of nausea and vomiting during transition. Another reason for limiting your food intake in early labor is that, should an emergency arise and you require general anesthesia, you could vomit and aspirate some of the liquid into your lungs. This could predispose you to pneumonia.

Your attendant will probably tell you to contact him when your contractions are seven to ten minutes apart. If they begin with an interval of five minutes, do not wait until the interval becomes greater, because it probably won't. Contractions come closer together as labor progresses. Also, the contractions may not be regular (although they usually are during labor).

Your attendant may tell you to call him when you think that the amniotic sac has broken. If you have any questions about what is happening, give him a call. Talk to him yourself rather than trying to use a third person. You should have available information about when the contractions began, how close they are, if and when your bag of waters broke, and any other symptoms you are having. He will give you instructions on what to do next.

WHAT TO TAKE TO THE HOSPITAL

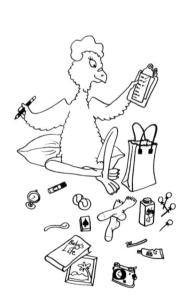

Your hospital stay should be as comfortable as possible, during labor and birth as well as your recovery period. The Lamaze Bag is designed to include items that you and your labor partner will use during labor and birth. Pack all of the suggested items, as you won't know which ones you will need until you go into labor. Pack items in your hospital bag that will personalize your hospital room. Hospital gowns are made for hospital patients, not for new mothers. Bringing your own gowns from home will also boost your spirits. Never pack items that are irreplaceable, such as jewelry or a great deal of money.

The Lamaze Bag

The Lamaze Bag should be kept apart from the suitcase, which will probably go to the postpartum room, rather than the birthing area. Most of the items contained in the bag are not available in the hospital. Prepare for the possibility of early labor by assembling most of this Lamaze or "goody bag" a couple of weeks before your due date. It may be helpful to keep this bag in the car in case you are not at home when labor begins. You then won't have to run home to get these items before going to the hospital. This will only be important if labor progresses rapidly, but since you cannot know what the duration of your labor will be, be a good scout and be prepared.

The contents of the Lamaze Bag should include items for all situations that may occur during labor:

For dry mouth:
- Breath spray, sour lollipops, gum, or a small cosmetic sponge to suck on.

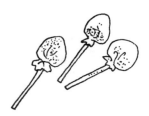

For dry lips:
- Vaseline petroleum jelly, Chap Stick lip balm, or lip gloss.

For effleurage:
- Talcum powder, lotion, or cornstarch.

For backache:
- Tennis balls or cold oranges.
- Athletic ice pack, Pringle's potato chips can, tennis ball can, or Tupperware rolling pin.
- Hot water bag or chemical heat.

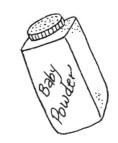

For labor in general:
- Socks to keep your feet warm and prevent trembling.
- Washcloth to refresh you when you are hot and sweaty.
- Small paper bag for hyperventilation.
- Object on which to concentrate, such as picture of baby, pair of booties, or something else that will remind you of your purpose.
- Pencil and paper for note taking.
- Stopwatch (if you have one).
- Sandwiches for labor partner (may be made and frozen in advance).
- Something for labor partner to drink.
- Safety pin in case the partner's scrub suit is very large and has no drawstring.
- Hand-held fan.
- Pillows (something from home for your comfort).
- Change for phone and list of phone numbers.

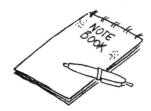

For mementos:
- Camera with film.
- Tape recorder (battery operated).

The Hospital Suitcase

During your hospital stay, most necessary equipment will be supplied for you. This will include hospital gowns, soap, sanitary napkins and belt, washcloths, towels, lotion, and a spray bottle for perineal hygiene. Any other item that you wish to have with you for your hygiene or comfort will have to be taken from home. You should bring the following:

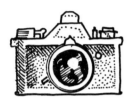

- Nightgowns or pajamas.
- Robe and slippers.
- Underwear (bra and panties).
- Toothbrush and toothpaste.
- Comb and brush.
- Shampoo and conditioner.
- Cosmetics.

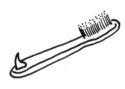

Some optional items you might consider taking are:

- Curling iron and/or blow dryer.
- Perfume.
- Favorite soaps, powders, or lotions.

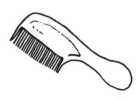

You may prefer beltless sanitary pads to the belt and pads supplied. If so, you will want to purchase a large box of the maxi or super-absorbent pads. If you use a sanitary belt, you may wish to bring an extra belt so that you will have a clean change if one gets soiled.

If you are planning to nurse your baby, you should bring nursing bras. Ideally, these should be purchased toward the end of the pregnancy. You may require a different cup size as nursing proceeds and your breasts adjust to the demands of the baby. You might also consider purchasing nursing gowns or gowns that can be easily and discreetly moved aside for nursing.

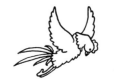

You may plan to bring something to keep you occupied while you are in the hospital and your baby is sleeping. Many women take their birth announcements to the hospital and fill them out there. You might also consider taking good books or handiwork.

Pack your suitcase well in advance to save a mad rush when labor starts. Have ready or pack an outfit for the baby to come home in, as well as one for yourself. Plan to wear an outfit that you wore during the middle of your pregnancy. Your beautiful figure will not return for several weeks, so be prepared to wear something loose for your comfort.

HOSPITAL ADMISSION ROUTINES

If possible, tour the labor and birthing area of your hospital several weeks before you are to be admitted. You will feel more relaxed and confident if you are familiar with the environment, procedures, and staff before you arrive. If your hospital allows preregistration, fill out the necessary papers before your due date. This may prevent a long delay for you and your partner.

When you arrive at the hospital for admittance, you will probably use the emergency room entrance. From there you will be taken to the labor and birth area in a wheelchair, which may make you feel silly because you will not feel sick. Your partner will probably be sent to register you if you have not done so already, and will then join you in the labor area. Meanwhile, you will be given a hospital gown to wear (a brief, original design from Paris). After you change, the nurse will ask you questions about your progress. If possible, answer these questions between contractions. She will then take your blood pressure, pulse, and temperature; listen to the baby's heartbeat; and time and assess the quality of your contractions. The procedures (except the temperature) will be repeated throughout labor, about every 15 to 30 minutes. You may have a vaginal examination to determine your progress. Relax your pelvic floor and use any breathing technique you feel necessary if the exam causes you discomfort.

In preparation for birth, the hair around the vaginal opening may be washed and cut. This is commonly referred to as a **"prep."** In the past, the pubic hair and all hair around the vagina and anus was shaved. This was called a "complete prep." Because it was often embarrassing and uncomfortable and its value in infection prevention has been questioned, many birth attendants now suggest that a "mini" or "partial" prep be done. This includes clipping the longer pubic hair and washing the vaginal and anal openings with an antiseptic soap. Sometimes the hair around the anus and vagina is shaved. Some women do not have any prep. This depends upon your

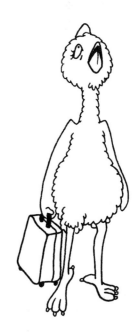

"Couldn't we just take the car?"

preferences and those of your birth attendant. Discuss this procedure with him during your pregnancy.

In preparation for labor, you may also be given an enema. If you have had a recent bowel movement or diarrhea, the rectum is probably already empty. If not, and if you are not well advanced into labor, your birth attendant may suggest an enema, as the fear of expelling feces during birth occasionally prevents a mother from pushing well. During the enema, lie on your left side with your upper leg flexed. You should consciously relax and use whatever techniques you feel are appropriate to ease discomfort. If your bag of waters has broken, you will probably use the bedpan; otherwise you will go to the bathroom to expel the enema. Once the bag of waters has broken, many birth attendants prefer that the mother not walk around. If the baby is high in the pelvis and has not engaged, there is a possibility that the umbilical cord will drop below the baby's head. This is a problem, because the cord then becomes compressed as the baby descends, thus clamping off the blood supply from the placenta. If the baby has already engaged, this is usually not a problem.

You will have vaginal examinations periodically, depending on the apparent progress of your labor. During these exams, remember to relax your pelvic floor and to use whatever techniques you feel are necessary. You may be asked to lie on your back for the exams, because they are otherwise difficult to perform. This may be uncomfortable and cause a backache. If so, employ the techniques described on pages 90–94, and get into a comfortable position again as soon as you can.

Before birth, your baby's heartbeat is a valuable indication of how he is reacting to labor. Because of this, the nurse or birth attendant will check the baby's heart rate after contractions, usually every 15 to 30 minutes. This monitoring may be done with a stethoscope, a fetoscope (a stethoscope with a headpiece), or a Doptone, which uses ultrasound waves to pick up the baby's heart rate. If there is a medical indication or reason to suspect that your baby may have some trouble during strong labor, e.g., diabetes, toxemia, or an erratic fetal heartbeat, a machine may be used to continuously monitor the baby. In some hospitals, continuous monitoring is used on all women in labor. See pages 101–105 for a discussion of electronic fetal monitoring.

THE PHYSICAL PROCESS OF CHILDBIRTH

Childbirth is divided into three stages: labor, birth, and afterbirth. The first stage extends from the beginning of labor until the cervix is completely dilated. The initial part of this stage is called the **early, preliminary,** or **effacement phase,** and lasts from the beginning of labor until the cervix is **dilated**, or opened, about 3 cm. During this phase the cervix also **effaces**, or shortens, and merges into the body of the uterus. The degree of effacement is expressed in percentages, with 100 percent effacement indicating complete cervical effacement. The cervix effaces approximately 70 to 80 percent during this phase of labor. Some effacement and dilation occur in the last month of pregnancy, before labor actually begins.

The second phase of labor is the **accelerated, active,** or **dilation phase**. The cervix dilates, or opens, to about 6 cm and finishes effacing during this time.

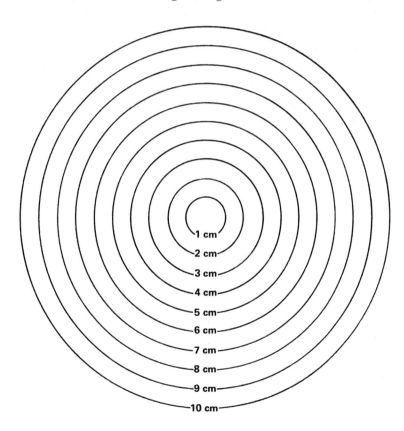

1 cm
2 cm
3 cm
4 cm
5 cm
6 cm
7 cm
8 cm
9 cm
10 cm

Figure 3.1
Dilation Chart (actual size)
During labor, the cervix dilates to permit the baby to pass out of the uterus. Dilation is complete at 10 cm.

The end of the first stage is called **transition**, during which the cervix dilates from about 7 to 10 cm. This is the shortest and most intense part of labor. Full dilation is 10 cm, or about 4 inches in diameter. (See Figure 3.1 on page 69.)

Birth, the second stage of childbirth, begins when the cervix is completely dilated and ends with the birth of the baby. During this stage the baby is pushed out of the uterus, down the birth canal or vagina, and into the world.

The third stage is the birth of the placenta or "afterbirth." During this time contractions continue, causing the placenta to separate from the uterine wall so it can be expelled.

Most women who have not yet given birth think that all the contractions of childbirth are terribly hard and painful. This is simply not true. The contractions of the effacement phase of labor are small and friendly ones. Those of the birth are hard but rewarding, because you push with them, and those of the third stage are so mild that you may be completely unaware of them. Isn't that reassuring? But—there is always a catch, isn't there?—the contractions in the middle of labor are hard and require strong attention to technique and much work to stay relaxed. These contractions can be downright unfriendly.

The following description is an example of a textbook labor. Your labor may not be exactly like this, since every labor is different.

The Effacement Phase

The effacement phase averages 4 to 12 hours in duration. Contractions during this time are shallow waves of sensation that last about 30 to 45 seconds, with intervals of 5 to 20 minutes in length. Each interval is timed from the beginning of one contraction to the beginning of the next one. As labor progresses, the intervals shorten. By placing a hand lightly on the uterus, just above the navel, the contractions may be felt by the coach or nurse before the mother feels them within. This may be difficult for the inexperienced person to do, especially if the mother is lying on her side. If done, however, the mother may benefit from the advance warning.

Contractions are usually felt low in the abdomen behind the pubic bone, or all around the front, back, and sides. They feel similar to a "fire burn" or "Indian burn" that increases and decreases in intensity. Some contractions are felt in the lower back only. This back labor can be very uncomfortable. For techniques to relieve back labor, see pages 90–94. Between contractions you will have almost no sensation of discomfort. This is the time to rest.

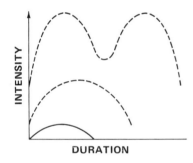

DURATION

Figure 3.2
The Effacement Contraction.
This diagram illustrates the 3 types of contractions you may experience during labor. The effacement contraction, which is emphasized here, is the least intense of the 3 types. Effacement contractions are usually 30–45 seconds in duration and come at 5–20 minute intervals.

Most of the 4 to 12 hours of the effacement phase will be spent at home in relative comfort, without the need for controlled breathing. When you can no longer talk normally through your contractions, begin using your techniques. You should not begin earlier, because you may tire or get discouraged. This is very important to remember, because although you may be excited and eager for labor to start, you may need to conserve your energy.

When you feel the need to do something during contractions, begin with slow deep breathing. With the slow, deep breathing you should perform effleurage, or light abdominal stroking, to release the superficial muscles, give you something to do with your hands, and increase the level of activity in your brain.

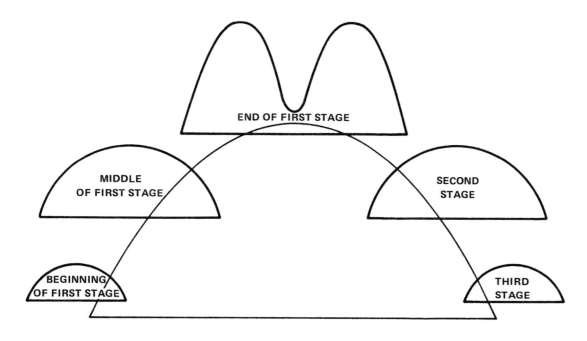

END OF FIRST STAGE

MIDDLE
OF FIRST STAGE

SECOND
STAGE

BEGINNING
OF FIRST STAGE

THIRD
STAGE

Figure 3.3
The Stages of Labor
Labor is at its most intense at the end of the first stage, during transition. After transition, you will move into the exhilarating second stage of birth.

Your brain activity can be further increased by mental concentration. Analyze the quality of each contraction as it rises to its peak and tapers off so that you can better determine your response. With each contraction, you should relax and breathe appropriately for the intensity you are experiencing. As the intensity increases you should increase the rate of your breathing, and as the contraction recedes you should slow your breathing. Some women find their concentration enhanced by opening their eyes and fixing them on a distant object. Others believe that they can relax and concentrate better with their eyes closed. Whichever method you choose, do not allow yourself to become distracted.

The Dilation Phase

The dilation phase averages 2 to 6 hours in duration. The contractions may last from 45 to 60 seconds, with intervals of 2 to 4 minutes in length. They are stronger and more regular than those of the first phase. They still begin gradually, but reach a higher peak of intensity and remain there longer before tapering off again. (See Figure 3.4.) During this period of labor, the effacement of the cervix may be completed, and you may dilate to about 6 cm.

To maintain control of the stronger contractions during the middle of labor, you will probably need to change to rapid shallow breathing. This breathing is shallow to provide the minimum amount of movement from the diaphragm, and rapid to provide you with the additional oxygen your working uterus needs. A long-distance runner learns how to adjust his breathing to the needs of his body to bring in more oxygen and to rid his body of the excess carbon dioxide. You, too, will need to adjust your breathing to your body's needs. During labor you will accelerate and decelerate your breathing rate as the contraction builds up and tapers off. You will continue to use the slow effleurage with the shallow breathing throughout labor.

Dilation is a long, difficult part of labor, and progress may seem slow. You may reach a plateau at which strong contractions continue but no dilation or effacement takes place. Try not to get discouraged. Once you get beyond this plateau, labor will progress nicely. During the dilation phase, you will realize that labor really does mean hard work.

Transition

The hard work becomes harder. Maximum effort is required to stay above transition contractions.

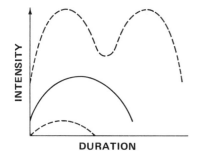

Figure 3.4
The Dilation Contraction
This contraction begins with greater intensity than the effacement contraction, reaches a higher peak, and lasts longer. Normally, these contractions are 45–60 seconds in duration and come at 2–4 minute intervals.

These contractions may last up to 90 seconds and may come every 1½ to 3 minutes. Because they are so close together, you will feel that you have no time to rest. Some of the contractions will be short and mild, but others will be the strongest you will ever encounter. These erratic contractions are difficult to deal with because you cannot plan your response to them. Begin your techniques with each contraction, even if you think that the contraction will be easy. It may not be the mild one you expected.

The character of the contractions changes now. They peak rapidly and may have more than one peak per contraction. Just when you think the contraction is going away, it may begin to peak again. (See Figure 3.5.) Many women feel that their contractions come one on top of another, when in reality the second contraction is a continuation of the first. Effacement is complete, and the dilation from 7 to 10 cm goes very rapidly. The contractions are hardest right before complete dilation.

There are two good things about transition (and only two). First, this phase usually lasts only 10 to 60 minutes, with an average of 30 minutes. It is the shortest phase of labor. The second encouraging fact is that once in transition, the birth of your baby is very near, and you will soon be in the second stage of labor: birth. You can then begin pushing, and pushing usually feels good. Keep that in mind, and take one contraction at a time.

As labor progresses, the baby descends lower into the pelvis. During transition this descent may produce several symptoms. The baby may put pressure on the blood vessels in the pelvic region, thus decreasing the circulation from your legs to your body. This may produce cramps in your calves or a dull ache in your thighs. For leg cramps, stretch the muscles by straightening the knee and pulling your foot toward your knee. To relieve aching thighs, have your partner "milk" the blood back to your body by firmly massaging your thigh from the knee down and lightly back to the knee several times.

Another possible result of the baby's descent is a backache caused by the pressure of the baby on the sacrum. See pages 90–94 for techniques to relieve backache.

As rectal and pelvic pressure increases, you may feel the urge to bear down. You should not push until you are fully dilated, unless your birth attendant tells you to push. Blowing out repeatedly and rapidly will prevent you from forcefully bearing down during this time. After each exhalation, you will automatically inhale. The blowing actually produces a slight pushing effect with the abdominal muscles, thus relieving the urge to push, while the following quick inhalation prevents you from bearing down.

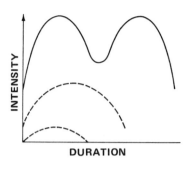

Figure 3.5
The Transition Contraction
These contractions intensify rapidly and often have more than one peak. They are 60–90 seconds in duration and come at 1½–3 minute intervals.

This rapid breathing may produce **hyperventilation**, which is caused by exhaling too much carbon dioxide. Another cause of hyperventilation is breathing too rapidly or deeply. Because the symptoms of hyperventilation are uncomfortable and may impair your ability to relax, you and your partner should watch for them. These symptoms include blurred vision, dizziness, and cramping in fingers and toes. You may also look "glassy-eyed." Fortunately, the symptoms can be easily corrected by rebreathing your own carbon dioxide. Cover your nose and mouth with either the bed sheet, your cupped hands, a surgical mask, or a paper bag, while you breathe in and out during contractions. Between contractions, simply hold your breath for a few seconds longer.

The symptoms of transition that result from your central nervous system's response to the stress of labor are not easily relieved. These symptoms include hot and cold flashes, trembling, nausea, vomiting, and hiccoughing. **Hot and cold flashes** are relieved by taking off or putting on more blankets. **Trembling**, although not due to cold, is relieved by extra blankets, especially around the feet. This warmth eventually stops the shivering, but until then you should not try to stop trembling by tensing up. It will not help. If someone holds your arms or legs or lightly strokes your inner thighs, it may provide some relief. Taking slow deep breaths between contractions may also help. **Nausea** may be relieved by a cool cloth placed on your face and neck, swallowing, and slow deep breathing between contractions. Avoid eating large quantities of food at the beginning of labor because digestion stops during labor. Vomiting a large amount of undigested or partially digested food can be very unpleasant.

Symptoms of transition that are due to the physical progress of labor include the progressive loss of the mucous plug, the breaking of the amniotic sac (if it has not already broken), exhaustion, irritability, and restlessness.

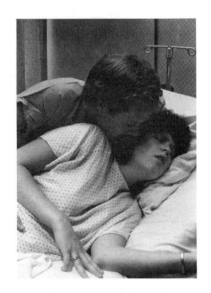

By the end of labor, the mother is tired.

As labor progresses and the cervix gradually dilates, the mucous plug, which closed the cervix during the pregnancy, is loosened. Sometimes this plug is released before labor begins, but more often it comes out during labor. As the cervix dilates, small blood vessels in the cervix may break and tinge the mucous discharge with blood. You will have an increase in the mucous "show," or "bloody show," during transition.

Although the bag of waters sometimes breaks before labor, it more often ruptures during transition due to the increased strength of the contractions and the pressure from the baby's head. This usually causes the uterine contractions to grow stronger, because as the amniotic fluid is released, the uterus can become smaller with each contraction. The more compact the uterus is, the stronger the contractions are. For this reason, the first or second contraction after the bag of waters breaks may feel significantly stronger than those before. Keep this in mind, and anticipate stronger contractions. You will probably be required to stay in bed after the membranes rupture.

Exhaustion, irritability, and restlessness are probably the most universal symptoms of transition, but none is specific to transition. These symptoms may occur individually at any time during labor, but when they occur together it may be a sign that the end of labor is near. During transition contractions, you may feel restless and be unable to find a comfortable position. Because the contractions are so close together, you may have only 15 to 30 seconds rest between them. No wonder you'll feel tired and irritable! Sometimes, however, you may forget your discomfort and fall sound asleep. This peculiar combination of restlessness during contractions and sleep between contractions is often specific to the latter part of transition.

You will not have all of these symptoms at once. They are listed primarily so that you will not be caught unaware if they should occur. Look for and recognize these symptoms so that you can determine when you are in transition.

If your partner notices that you are becoming restless and fatigued, he should suggest that you change your position, wipe your forehead and neck with a cool washcloth, and hold you closely during contractions or maintain some physical or visual contact with you. He should offer as much support as possible, reminding you that labor is almost over and that your baby will soon be born. He should also be ready to have his efforts impatiently rebuffed. Remember that this is transition, and that transition often creates irritability.

Caution: Once you begin to experience any of these symptoms you are probably in transition, regardless of how far dilation has progressed. The dilation of the cervix may lag behind the intensity of the contractions, but it will soon catch up. Remember, once you are in transition, the unpleasant part of labor is almost over.

During transition, internal examinations to determine the progress of labor are more frequent. Your perineal area may be cleansed with an antiseptic before the exam. Make sure that you relax your pelvic floor, or the examination will be very uncomfortable. You may need to utilize your breathing techniques at this time.

During transition you will usually use a pant-blow, or pattern paced, breathing, even if you have no desire to push. This breathing requires greater concentration, and will therefore increase the level of mental activity. You will probably not want to perform the effleurage yourself at this time as it may make you tense instead of relaxing you, so rest your arms comfortably, or use

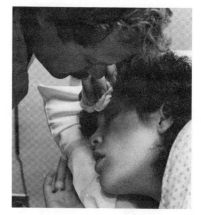

The labor partner's loving support is important. Here, the partner uses a cool cloth to soothe and refresh the mother.

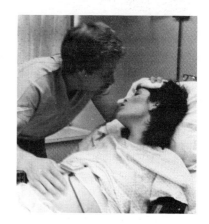

During transition, the labor partner often assumes the responsibility of performing effleurage.

them to support your uterus. Your partner should practice effleurage in advance so that he can assume this responsibility during transition if you desire it.

Remember that transition is the shortest part of labor, and that *labor will not get harder.* Do not expect transition to be painless. There may be pain, but the pain won't be unbearable, and you will be able to control it to a great extent with your Lamaze techniques. When you are fully dilated, you will be able to push, and pushing is usually exhilarating and pleasant.

The Second Stage of Childbirth

This stage begins with full dilation (10 cm) and ends with the birth of the baby. When the cervix is completely open, the baby leaves the uterus. He does not pull and push to get himself born; he is a passive passenger in the birth canal. Because he is wet and slippery, he does not stick anywhere as the mother bears down. His body adjusts and turns to move down the birth canal, just as your body would adjust to the curves in the circular "tornado" sliding board at the park. His mother pushes him out. As he descends, the baby turns so that the widest dimension of his head (from front to back) enters the widest part of the mother's pelvis.

The baby enters the pelvis facing his mother's side, and rotates about 45 degrees to face her back at the ischial spines. He then pivots under the pubic bone and crowns. Crowning occurs when the top of the baby's head (the occiput) is visible at the vaginal opening (+4 station). After his head is born, he rotates again to face the mother's thigh, thus allowing the shoulders to pass under the pubic bone and emerge, one shoulder at a time. The rest of the body then slips out easily.

This is what happens to your baby within. But what will be happening to you, and how will you feel?

During birth, the contractions are like those of the dilation phase, lasting 40 to 60 seconds, with one peak per contraction. The interval between contractions lengthens to 3 to 7 minutes, giving you a chance to rest between them. During this stage of labor, you will be pushing with each contraction unless you are told not to push. As your baby's head is being born, your attendant may tell you to stop pushing so that the birth can be gentle and guided. To do this you must release all your muscles, lie back gently, exhale, and do the shallow breathing employed during dilation. This requires some advance practice.

You will be surprised by how quickly this stage passes. If this is your first baby, you will probably push for approximately 20 to 30 minutes to bring your baby to crowning. You will then

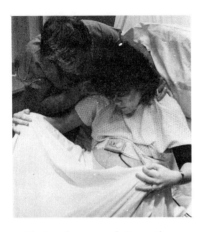

During the second stage of labor, the mother pushes the baby down the birth canal.

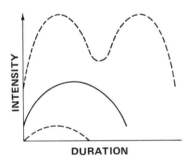

Figure 3.6
The Birth Contraction
The contractions of birth are similar to those of the dilation phase. They are usually 40–60 seconds in duration and come at 3–7 minute intervals.

be moved into the delivery room, where you will push for another 15 to 20 minutes to deliver your baby.

If you have already had a baby, you will probably push for a shorter period of time, as your vagina and pelvic floor have already been stretched. Your transfer to the delivery room will most likely take place during transition or shortly thereafter, and all of your pushing will be done in that room.

Birth is the most satisfying stage of labor. During labor, all you can do is relax and not interfere with the uterus. During birth, you can actively work to give birth to your baby. You will be tired after each contraction, but pushing usually feels good.

Many women think that birth is the most painful part of labor, and if you do not relax your pelvic floor, it will be. If you relax your pelvic floor, the sensations of birth will be pleasant. If birth is not painful, what does it feel like?

With your first few pushes, you will probably feel that nothing is happening, as the baby will still be within the pelvis at that time. As he descends and enters the muscular vagina, you will begin to feel a build-up of pressure. When your baby starts to dilate the vaginal opening, you will feel a burning, stretching sensation, followed by numbness. This natural anesthesia is produced by the pressure from the baby's head, which compresses the blood vessels that supply the nerves in the area. The actual birth will be felt as a sliding sensation, a lessening of great pressure, and finally a warmth outside you, either from your baby brushing you or from the amniotic fluid that follows. You will be amazed by how quickly birth is over!

What about the **episiotomy**? This is an incision made to enlarge the vaginal opening. Your attendant will decide whether or not to perform this procedure at the time of birth. Many physicians believe that the tissues of the perineum will usually stretch for birth, while others perform the episiotomy routinely.

Several things can be done to increase the elasticity of the vaginal opening. During birth, good pelvic floor muscle tone can help to speed the dilation of the perineum. Pelvic muscle tone can be greatly improved by practicing the Kegel exercises frequently throughout pregnancy. (See pages 33–34.)

The mother's position for pushing is another factor that affects the pelvic floor. Women in many parts of the world squat for birth. Others assume a reclining squat, which is essentially the same position, except that the mother leans back against another person or against pillows at about a 45 to 60 degree angle, with her legs flexed and comfortably apart. This position allows for greater expansion of the pelvis and less stress on the perineum. Other women give birth in a side-lying position.

The pushing technique, also, affects the pelvic floor. If the mother pushes constantly during the birth contractions, the baby will move down the birth canal more quickly. In some cases this is desirable. If the mother pushes only when she feels the urge to bear down, the baby will descend more slowly, which may give the perineum more time to stretch. When birth is imminent, the birth attendant may massage the perineum or apply warm compresses to facilitate the thinning and stretching process. Be sure to discuss the issues of birth positions, pushing methods, and the episiotomy with your attendant well before your due date.

As your baby's head emerges, the perineum will stretch considerably. Occasionally, it appears that the vaginal opening is not stretching fast enough, and that there is a possibility of a tear. If a tear appears imminent, your birth attendant will do an episiotomy to prevent it. Both the depth and direction of the opening can be controlled by performing an episiotomy.

If an episiotomy is performed, you will not feel the incision because of the natural anesthesia of birth. You may feel as if a very tight pair of jeans or slacks has been unzipped. A local anesthetic may be given either before or after the baby is born, so that you will not be able to feel the repair after your natural anesthesia has worn off. If an episiotomy is not performed, you will feel the stretching and burning sensation of birth longer, because the perineum will dilate more.

The rest of your baby will be born in one or two contractions. Right after the head is born, the birth attendant will check to see if the cord is around the baby's neck. If it is, the attendant will elect to either clamp and cut it or push it aside. Mucus will be suctioned from the baby's nose and mouth to clear the breathing passages. Your baby may cry right away, or may start crying a few minutes after birth.

Do not be shocked by your baby's appearance. He will look very different after he has been bathed and dried, but directly after birth he will probably look blue, wet, and puffy. He may be covered with a cheesy substance called **vernix**, which protected his delicate skin while he was in the womb. He may also have some bloody fluid on his body from the birth passage. His color will be blue until he has been breathing on his own for a few minutes. His face may be puffy and his skin wrinkled, as if he has been soaking in water (which he has been for nine months). The genitals may be large due to maternal hormones; this, also, is temporary.

Your baby's head may be elongated as a result of **molding** during passage down the birth canal. This, too, will disappear in a few days. The bones of the baby's skull are not firmly

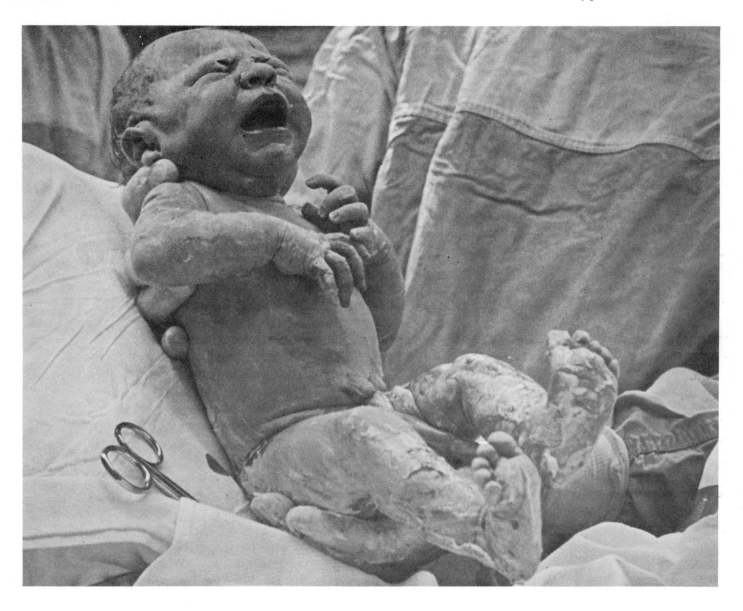

connected so that they can overlap during birth, enabling the baby's head to conform to the contours of the birth passage. Pointed head and all, he will probably look beautiful to you, and his first sounds will be music to your ears.

The Third Stage of Childbirth: Afterbirth

After birth, the contractions will be very mild, similar to those of early labor. You may not be aware of them at all. So many things will be happening! The attendant will continue to suction mucus from your baby's nose and mouth. The cord will be clamped and cut, which neither you nor your baby will feel, as there are no nerves in the cord. As you examine every detail of your beautiful baby, he may cry to let you know that he has arrived. But still the contractions will continue, because labor will not yet be over.

You may be given a hormone injection to assist the uterus in contracting, thus preventing excessive bleeding after the delivery of the placenta. These uterine contractions will cause the placenta to separate and drop to the base of the uterus. The separated placenta is usually delivered by the combined efforts of you and your birth attendant. As you push, the attendant will lift it out by placing tension on the cord. Some blood will be expelled with the placenta. Your attendant will then perform a thorough examination to insure that there are no fragments of the placenta or the bag of waters inside. He will also check for internal tears. When he has completed the examination, he will repair the episiotomy if one was performed. If you have any discomfort during the third stage of labor, relax your pelvic floor and use the slow deep or shallow breathing techniques as you feel the need.

During this time, the nurse will dry your baby and will either give him to you or your partner to hold next to your warm body, or place him in a heated crib to help him adjust to the drastic temperature change (98.6 degrees *in utero* to 70 degrees in the delivery room). Before you and your baby leave the birthing area, he will have identification bands placed on his wrist and ankle with the same number and name as the one placed on your arm. You will probably feel tired but quite exhilarated.

You may either stay in the birthing area or go to an observation room for a couple of hours. The staff will perform frequent checks of your blood pressure and pulse, and will examine your vaginal discharge and uterus. These examinations are done to monitor and prevent excessive bleeding and other medical problems. The uterus must contract and close off the blood vessels that supplied the placenta. If you are uncomfortable when your abdomen is being checked, release your muscles and do whatever breathing technique you feel necessary. Have the nurse tell you before she begins to check your abdomen, so that you can be ready with your techniques. You may also have ice packs applied to your abdomen and perineum to aid the uterine contractions and prevent swelling of the episiotomy site.

Many women experience trembling after their baby's birth. Warmth, gentle restraint, and slow deep breathing may relieve this trembling. You should urinate soon after birth to prevent discomfort from a distended bladder. If you have trouble doing this, contract and release your pelvic floor several times and whistle a tune as you sit on the toilet or bedpan. These techniques will enable you to urinate more easily.

Another word about episiotomies. You will be able to walk normally soon after birth and avoid the "episiotomy shuffle" if you begin your pelvic floor exercises (Kegels) in the recovery area and continue doing them often during the first few weeks after birth. These exercises will help the episiotomy heal faster and markedly decrease discomfort. If you are uncomfortable sitting, do not use a pillow or rubber ring. These will put tension on your stitches and make them hurt more. Instead, squeeze your buttocks together before sitting on a firm surface and release your buttocks after you are seated. The one and only drawback of Lamaze preparation is that you may have difficulty sleeping after birth. You will be tired, but too excited to sleep as you relive your fantastic birth experience. Use your relaxation exercises and slow deep breathing to help yourself sleep.

THE POSTPARTUM PERIOD

The term **postpartum** is used to describe the first six weeks after the birth of a baby. During this time the uterus shrinks in weight from two pounds to two ounces. This process is called **involution**.

During the postpartum period you will have a vaginal discharge called **lochia**. Lochia, which is present for three to four weeks, is the product of the cleansing and healing process that takes place in the uterus after childbirth. This discharge, which is composed of blood, tissue, and mucus, will initially be bright red. After several days, the discharge will become watery and pink. This will last from three to ten days. You will then notice the discharge clearing and thinning. The lochia usually disappears around the third week, although some brown spotting may persist for a few more days. Fresh bleeding that occurs after the discharge has become slight should be reported to your doctor. You may notice an increase in the amount of lochia if you overexert yourself. It is important to rest during the first weeks after birth.

During the first few days after birth, you may experience noticeable contractions. These contractions will be intermittent, and are most likely to occur when you breastfeed your baby. The uterus will contract to close all the blood vessels that supplied the placenta during pregnancy and to help the uterus return to its normal state. These contractions are not too noticeable after first babies, but are more common after subsequent children. If they are uncomfortable, you should respond as you did to the labor contractions—with specific breathing and relaxation techniques.

If you do not breastfeed, you will probably menstruate within eight weeks after birth. If you do breastfeed, menstruation may be delayed for four to eighteen months, because there is usually no ovulation during lactation. (Be aware that exceptions have occurred, and be sure to use some method of birth control, unless you want your babies' birthdays to fall very close together!)

Your body will have a lot of adjusting to do after birth, so take care of yourself during the postpartum period. Get plenty of rest, keep your perineum clean, and do the exercises your birth attendant prescribes. This should be a pleasant time for your new family.

THE EMOTIONAL ASPECTS OF CHILDBIRTH

Early Labor

For many of you, childbirth will be one of the most highly charged emotional events of your life. When labor begins, you will experience not only physical changes, but very strong emotional changes as well. When the first contractions of labor begin, you may feel a combination of excitement, happiness, and, perhaps, a sense of relief that the waiting is over. This is the fun time of labor. The contractions will be mild and you will feel happy. No more waiting! No more urinating every half hour! You will soon be able to sleep comfortably, wear nice clothes, walk, run, sit, stand, and jump easily. Best of all, you will soon hold and cuddle your new baby. You've waited a long time for this! Everyone will want to wait on you. Let them. Do not waste time cleaning the house or preparing meals. Enjoy yourself. All too soon this phase will be over and you will be immersed in the work phase of labor.

At some point in the beginning of labor you may also experience some apprehension, and possibly a brief moment of panic at the sudden realization that "this is it." Your partner should be aware of this possibility and help you to relax. Because you are armed with all the tools you need, you will be able to cope with the increasing strength of the contractions. Your preparation will help you to be calm and confident. You will soon realize that labor is hard work, and will become more intent upon your contractions and your response to them. At that point you should try to relax and allow yourself to flow with the process of labor. Trust your body.

Labor may be a lonely time for you, for you will be going where no one else can go with you or for you. This is the journey into motherhood and it is awesome, but it need not be frightening. You will be surrounded by those who love you and can help you—your partner, nurse, and birth attendant.

Transition

The need for closeness may arise as the strength of the contractions increases. Partners, you will have to get right next to the mother and talk into her face if you want to be heard. It may help if you encourage her to open her eyes and concentrate on your face during transition, rather than closing her eyes or focusing on some distant object or point. Many women claim to have received the strength to go on just by concentrating on their labor partners' eyes. You may try holding her. Some women reject physical contact at this point, while others need it. You will have to find out what she needs and wants. Do not feel personally rejected if she does not wish to be touched. This is not an uncommon reaction during transition.

As the mother approaches full dilation, the contractions will achieve their maximum strength and she will have reached what is referred to as the "emotional booby trap" of labor. You should understand some of the feelings she may encounter during this most rapid part of labor, because they can be very unpleasant. Many women express great irritability, either verbally or physically. If she appears angry, do not take this personally. She is angry at labor, not at you. This anger will pass when she begins pushing. Team effort will be required to help her until then. She may want to get away from labor. She may start inching toward the head of the bed ("I'll get up here and leave my uterus down there and then I'll be fine"), but when she moves, her uterus goes with her. She may say or think, "I want to go home now" ("This labor room is causing my contractions"), or she may go into a deep sleep ("I'll just sleep here until it's time to push"), but

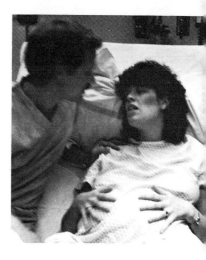

Eye contact may give the mother the feeling of closeness and support that she needs.

the contractions wake her up. She may ask for pain medication ("Give me a shot and put me to sleep"). Medication will help her to sleep between contractions, but she will still awaken for the contractions. Usually, when a mother asks for medication, she is nearing the completion of labor. Often the mother doesn't realize this, and thinks that she has several more hours to go before birth. Once dilated she will be able to push, and won't want to get away from labor anymore.

One of the biggest problems that faces the mother in advanced labor is fear—fear that she will "not be able to stand it" if the contractions get stronger. However, many women who have taken medication in a moment of panic have been disappointed afterwards, and have said that if they had only known how close they were to complete dilation, they would not have taken the medication. Often just knowing that the end of labor is near relieves the mother's fear, enabling her to go on. If the mother indicates that she wants medication, you should find out if the contraction she just had was very painful, or if she is fearful about future contractions. You should encourage her to take one contraction at a time. Once transition contractions begin, they do not get stronger. If she can handle one, she can probably handle them all, one at a time. If you have reason to suspect that she is in transition, inform her of this. Often, progress has been made since the last examination. It may help her to be told how far dilated she is.

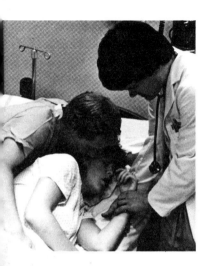

Team effort is especially important during transition. The mother should be surrounded by those who care.

Throughout labor, you may be able to identify the mother's progress by observing her behavior. During early labor, she will probably be excited, fairly talkative, and comfortable. Her conversation will be about many different things. If you ask her how she is doing, she will probably happily answer, "Oh fine, the contractions aren't hard. No trouble at all."

As labor progresses it will be apparent to everyone that the mother is working harder with the contractions. Discussion will now be about the labor, how the baby is doing, and how much longer it will be until birth. Ask her now how she is doing, and she will wearily reply, "Oh . . . okay, but this is really hard."

At the end of labor, during the transition phase, the mother will be concentrating completely on labor, and will often appear very tired or restless. She may have one or more of the symptoms of transition discussed earlier. If she responds at all to questions it will be with grunts or one-word answers. She will not usually initiate a conversation except to ask "How much longer?" or to complain. If you ask how she is feeling, she may respond with a growl, profanity, silence, or "Oh, shut up!"

Many women have an image of what they think is the perfect labor patient—quiet, relaxed, controlled, and maybe even smiling. Often women who value their self-control and independence are terrified of losing control in labor and embarrassing themselves. It is time to recognize that birth is a part of a woman's life, and as such is subject to the same feelings and reactions that occur daily. During labor and birth, the mother will not become a different person. She will still be herself. If when frustrated, irritated, apprehensive, and in pain, she responds by being quiet, relaxed, and controlled—and maybe even smiling—she will probably do so in labor. But if she responds to frustration, irritation, apprehension, and pain with tears or anger, she will probably do so in labor, because all of these factors will be present in labor.

If after a hard day's work your wife came home frustrated and irritated and then tripped and sprained her ankle, you would not respond by offering her morphine and telling her not to be such a baby. You would probably respond with caring words, caresses, massage, and an icepack for her ankle. The same type of response will work well in labor. Partners and birth attendants must allow women to be themselves without feeling guilty or ashamed. The partner and birth attendant also must not feel that they have done a poor job if the mother reacts with tears or anger.

Believe it or not, when the symptoms of transition occur, everyone should rejoice. A definite milestone has been reached, indicating that the first stage is almost over.

Birth

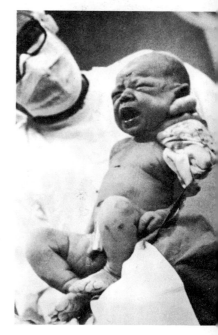

The newborn baby is presented to the world.

Excitement often accompanies the second stage of childbirth. As your baby's head comes into view, everyone will become excited. You will be the star performer, with all present cheering you on. Leave your modesty at the door of the birthing area. You may claim it again after your baby is born. Because pushing demands strenuous effort, you will feel tired. But your exhilaration will allow you to respond with increasing vigor to your body's powerful need to push. Many women do not think about having a baby while they are pushing, but have a determination to "push it out of there." Right before your baby is born, you may feel the sudden realization that there is no way to escape. You are about to become a mother! Before you have time to digest that thought, your baby will be born.

A tremendous feeling of relief will follow. Not relief from pain, but from extremely hard, physical labor. Do not let anyone tell you that there is no work involved in having a baby! You will feel a rush of pride and awe as you examine your new baby and listen to him cry. You and your partner will both feel tired but elated and proud of your participation in the miracle that is birth.

The Leboyer Method

Besides the emotional aspects of childbirth for the parents, some consideration has recently been given to the effect of childbirth on the baby. For years, all anyone wanted was a physically healthy and crying baby. Dr. Frederick Leboyer, author of *Birth Without Violence*, implores us to look at birth from the child's point of view. Contractions compress him, finally pushing him down a narrow tube and out into a cold, bright world. He is wrapped in a dry, prickly cloth and placed on a flat surface, cold and alone. What an introduction to life outside the uterus!

With very few modifications, birth can be made more pleasant for your baby. The lights in the birthing area can be dimmed, with only the perineum spotlighted to allow the birth attendant to see what is going on. Prior to this, the baby experienced nothing but darkness (unless someone has held a bright light to the mother's abdomen, which he sees as diffused shadows). Remember how it takes time for your eyes to adjust when going from a dark room into the bright sunlight?

Another slight modification can be made by keeping the baby's back rounded as he is born. Think of how you stretch in the morning after lying on your side at night. You would not feel comfortable suddenly straightening your back. The baby's back has been rounded since he started developing a spinal column at four weeks of age, and will therefore feel more comfortable if allowed to gradually move out of that position.

After birth, the baby can be placed on his side on the mother's abdomen. The mother's abdomen is soft—a real "jelly belly"—and moves gently as she breathes. While there, the mother can gently caress and explore her baby easily. She will probably do so tentatively at first, and later with more assurance. Thus will begin the love relationship between mother and child.

Leboyer also suggests that the first breath of air rushing into the lungs burns. If the cord is allowed to function until it stops pulsating on its own, Leboyer claims, the baby will continue to receive oxygen from the mother and will not have to suck air into his lungs to survive. He can then begin breathing gradually, without experiencing any burning sensation.

The next modification—silence at the time of birth—is advised by Leboyer because he feels that the newborn's hearing is very sensitive. He suggests that the sounds in the birthing area may seem loud and harsh to the newborn, who has previously only heard the muted sounds of his mother's heartbeat, and her body's gurgling and rumbling. Leboyer advocates hushed tones that will not startle the baby.

Leboyer also suggests that the newborn be bathed in warm water to provide a transition from the intrauterine life to the hospital environment. After he has been born and allowed to rest on his mother's abdomen for a while, the baby should be placed in body temperature water to help him relax. The water is soothing, soft, and caressing. The baby can look around quietly, gently kicking and stretching. He probably will not cry.

Many childbirth attendants have incorporated some of Leboyer's techniques into their routine procedures, but still have some reservations about adopting all of them. Controversy exists over a delay in cutting the cord. Some attendants are concerned that excess blood may be transfused into the baby. In cases such as Rh incompatibility or infant cardiac weakness, this delay would not be good for the baby.

Some birth attendants believe that silence at the moment of birth may produce unnecessary tension in the parents. The baby has never been in total silence. He has been listening to the sounds of his mother for months. Most often the sounds he hears are not loud, but sometimes mothers do yell. At the time of birth, many women make noise as they bear down, or call out with joy or relief as the baby is born. To impose total silence upon the mother and father at this moving moment may place a great burden on them.

The water bath may be technically difficult to provide because of the need for a basin and warm water set at body temperature. In addition, some attendants fear that bathing a baby in a cool room may cause him to chill, and may eventually result in respiratory problems. Experience does not seem to support this theory. Babies seem to stay warm when given the bath or gently rubbed with warm water.

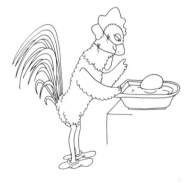

Some birth attendants feel uneasy having the lights dimmed. They are concerned about not being able to observe the mother's condition and the baby's color, which is an indication of his well-being.

If any of the Leboyer techniques appeal to you, discuss your feelings with your birth attendant at one of your prenatal visits. It is important to arrive at a mutually agreeable decision before labor begins. You are much more likely to get the kind of experience you want if you arrange for it in advance.

More than anything else, the techniques suggested by Frederick Leboyer provide a concrete way to change the attitude of everyone involved in the birth process, including the birth attendant, nursing staff, and parents. In this way, the techniques have been generally successful. Today, the goal of a healthy mother and baby has been expanded to include not just physical health, but mental and emotional health as well.

Chapter Four
Childbirth Variations

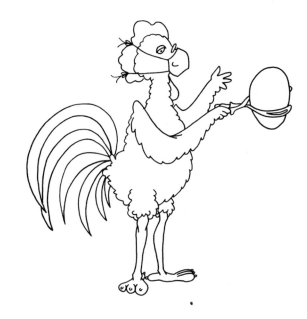

There are several factors that can make your childbirth experience different from the textbook description provided in the previous chapter. Your baby may be lying in a position that affects either your perception of the contractions or the progress of labor, or you may experience what is called a "plateau." In this situation, the contractions seem to be of good quality, but no progress in effacement or dilation occurs.

When these or any other variations occur, it may be necessary to make use of the medical technology that has been developed to monitor and assess the baby's condition. In addition, medical intervention may be necessary to assure a healthy baby and a healthy mother. The appropriate use of testing procedures, medications, and medical apparatus is the responsibility of the birth attendant and the pregnant woman. Well before your due date, discuss these topics with your birth attendant.

BACK LABOR

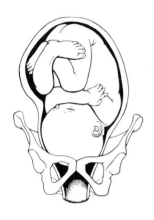

Figure 4.1
Posterior Presentation
In a posterior presentation, the back of the baby's head is pressed against the back of the uterus. Backache most commonly occurs when the baby's head is on the left side of the uterus.

You may experience backache during labor due to the position of the baby or the strain on the uterosacral ligaments which support the uterus. The baby usually lies in the right or left side of the pelvis with his head down, facing your spine. If, instead, he lies with the back of his head against your spine, he is in a **posterior position** (see Figure 4.1). You should prepare for this situation, since back labor can be very different from the textbook labor described earlier.

A posterior presentation may produce close, strong contractions that begin at the onset of labor. The pattern of the contractions may be somewhat erratic and unpredictable. They are most often perceived as a very severe backache, either at the waist or lower down at the sacrum. Unlike the typical labor, a dull, constant backache may linger between contractions. You may also experience aches in the thighs. To make childbirth even more challenging, the entire first stage may be prolonged. Most women do not have sufficient room in the lower portion of the pelvis to give birth to a baby who is in a posterior position. The baby who is in this position must rotate about 135 degrees for birth, rather than completing the 45 degree rotation of a baby who is in an anterior position (facing the spine). Labor contractions usually produce this rotation. As the baby rotates, you will probably notice a definite change in sensation. The backache will decrease in intensity, and you will gradually experience more discomfort in the lower abdominal area.

If your baby does not turn by the time you reach the second stage, you may still have a backache during birth. Your ability to push properly and cooperate fully may help the baby to rotate. Often the birth attendant will suggest that you push on your side or on all fours (hands and knees) to rotate the baby to a better position for birth. If a change of position doesn't cause the baby to rotate, the attendant will assist the birth by turning the baby with forceps.

The measures you take to handle the back labor situation are most important! You can do very well with this type of labor using your Lamaze techniques, but it will call for more effort from you and your partner. This is a time when your training together is so very important. Unless otherwise directed by your birth attendant or the nursing staff, follow these suggestions and adapt them to your own individual needs. Try as many as possible.

Labor Positions

You should assume a position that will favor the rotation of the baby and increase your comfort. The best position to assume in back labor is an all-fours position. Gravity will then help to bring the baby out of the posterior position and into an anterior one. Unfortunately, the all-fours position is uncomfortable, causing tension in the neck and shoulders. You can prevent this tension and achieve the same result by kneeling and resting your head and shoulders on the seat of a cushioned chair.

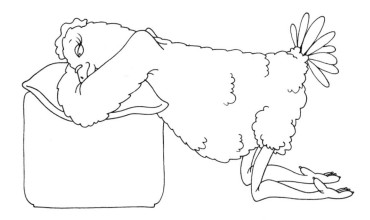

It may take quite a while to rotate the baby. If you experience contractions in your back during early labor, get into the modified all-fours position and stay there. Read, watch TV, talk to friends, and relax. In the hospital, you can kneel on your bed, leaning forward against the elevated head of the bed and covering your back with the sheet. While in a modified all-fours position, use the active pelvic rock either during or between contractions. Do this by arching your back upwards (as a cat stretches), causing your pubic bone to move forward and your abdominal muscles to tense slightly. Hold this position for a few seconds, then relax. *Caution:* Do not allow

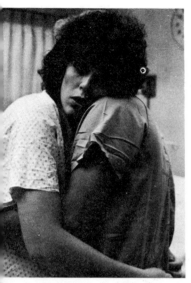

Walking or standing may help to ease backache.

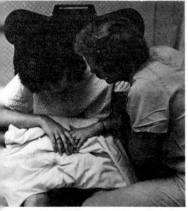

Backache can often be relieved by sitting in a chair with your back rounded.

yourself to get really swaybacked when you relax. Start with normal flexion, and round your back. The arching motion plus the force of gravity and the contractions may facilitate rotation.

Another position you can try is the side-lying position. Lie either with both legs and arms forward and bent comfortably, or with your lower leg straight, your upper leg flexed and supported by pillows, and your lower arm behind and alongside your back. These two positions will allow the weight of the baby to be carried by the bed, and not by your back.

You should also try walking and squatting during your back labor. This, too, will allow gravity to assist in the descent and rotation of the baby. During a labor in which you are experiencing a backache, change your position every half-hour. Move from the left side-lying position to the modified all-fours; change to the right side-lying position; and finally try standing, squatting, walking, or a semi-reclining position. Sitting in a chair with your back rounded, too, may increase your comfort. Many women appear reluctant to change their position once they get into active labor, and their partners have to encourage them to do so. Who knows? The new position may be more comfortable than the old one!

Counterpressure and Massage

Backache can sometimes be relieved by exerting pressure against the area of discomfort with the heel of the palm, fist, or thumb and fingertips. Aluminum cans that have been filled with water and frozen, tennis balls, or oranges may also be used. While applying pressure, your labor partner should prop his elbow against his hip and use his body for leverage to avoid fatigue and muscle strain. He should be careful not to exert too much pressure, as it can easily become painful rather than pain relieving. If you use frozen cans, your partner should place a washcloth around the can and then roll the can or press it into your back. If the frozen cans feel too cold, he should try exerting pressure with a cold washcloth.

When you are lying on your side, your partner can try massaging your back by supporting the upper hip and pressing the thumb and fingers of the other hand into your back. With the thumb in place, he should rotate the fingertips for a strong, localized massage. This procedure can be alternated with a gentle stroking of the back to aid in relaxation, which may become difficult because of the constant backache. The finger-pressure massage to the lower back area is very helpful and relaxing to these painful muscles. To prevent irritation, your partner's hands should be lubricated with lotion or baby powder before the massage.

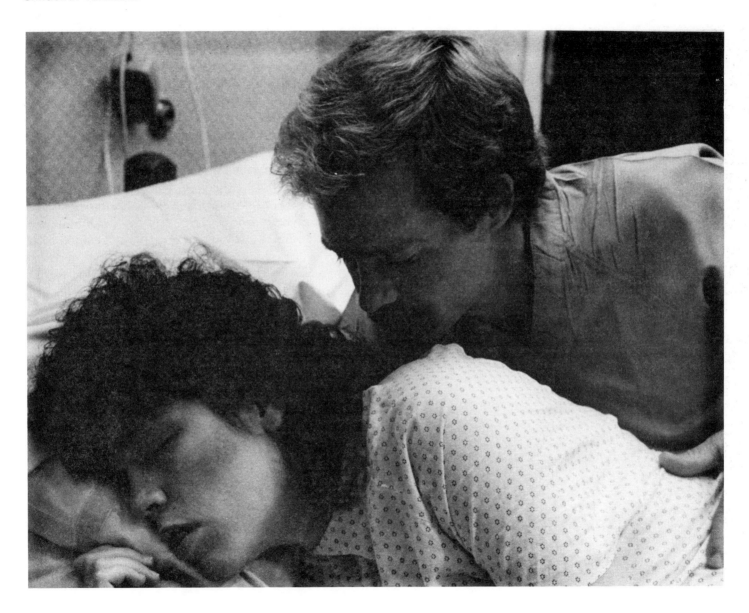

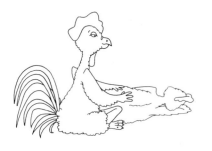

If your backache is due to strain on the uterosacral ligaments rather than the position of your baby, you may feel the contractions both in the front (under the pubic bone) and in the back. Although this backache will not be as severe as that experienced with a posterior position, you should use the same techniques for relief.

Do not underestimate the effort required to maintain control if you experience back labor. This is the most difficult type of labor. Practice techniques for the relief of back pain *thoroughly* in advance of labor. You will then have the basic tools with which to handle your sensations, and will be able to map out your own course of action to fit your individual labor. Rarely are two labors alike; each labor is different. It is essential that you and your partner work together in this situation. He should give constant encouragement, praise, and guidance. You may not obtain as much relief from your techniques as you would if the baby were in a more desirable position, but you will get results. You just have to work harder.

PLATEAUS

If you were to draw a chart depicting the progress of labor, you would notice that the first phase of labor (effacement) takes a long time, the second phase (dilation) goes more quickly, and the last phase (transition) passes very quickly. Plotting this "average" labor would result in a curve such as Line A in Figure 4.2.

Figure 4.2
Labor Progress
Line A represents the progress of most labors. In the labor described by Line B, a plateau occurs at 5 cm dilation.

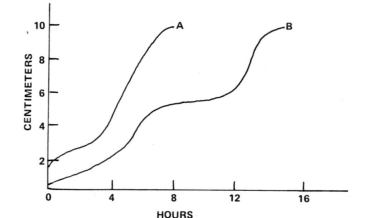

Frequently, labor does not follow this curve. Instead it may seem as if you are on a treadmill, working hard, but getting nowhere. Plotting such a labor on a chart would result in a curve like that shown in Figure 4.2, Line B. Note the plateau at 5 cm. Dilation appears to stop. This most often occurs before 5 cm, but can occur later.

Plateaus can be very discouraging. It may help to keep in mind that labor progress is measured in terms of three factors—effacement, dilation, and descent. You may not be dilating, but perhaps the cervix is thinning more, or the baby is being pushed lower into the pelvis. Assume that progress is occurring in one of these other areas. You will notice on Figure 4.2 that once a plateau is over, labor usually progresses very rapidly.

There are several possible causes for a plateau, or failure to progress. One cause may be a full bladder. Actually, the full bladder may produce a "true" and a "false" plateau. As you will note in Figure 2.3 (see page 18) there is not much room for the bladder as the baby moves into the pelvis. The uterus may put pressure on the full bladder during contractions and make you feel that you are having very strong contractions. In reality, you may be having very mild contractions and very strong bladder pressure and only be in the early part of labor, which goes slowly. This is a false plateau.

The full bladder may also present an obstacle to the baby's descent, producing a true plateau. As the baby descends lower into the pelvis, pressure from his head and the bag of waters dilates the cervix. This effect is decreased if the baby cannot get below the full bladder, thus prolonging labor. Avoid these situations by trying to urinate frequently—about once every hour—during labor. If you have trouble urinating, contract and release your pelvic floor several times, or whistle a tune. Whistling causes the abdominal muscles to be pushed downward and relaxes the pelvic floor, facilitating urination.

Another possible cause of a plateau is the position of the baby. In the discussion on posterior position, we pointed out that this position prolongs the dilation process, because the contractions usually have to push the baby into an anterior position before he can descend easily. If the baby's position causes you to reach a plateau, use the techniques described on pages 91–92 to aid the baby's rotation.

Your position, also, can affect your progress. During labor you assume positions that are comfortable for you, unless you are otherwise directed by the staff or your doctor. Try walking, standing, squatting, sitting in a chair, tailor-sitting in bed, lying on your back with the head and knee of the bed elevated, or lying on your left side. Avoid lying flat on your back, because the heavy uterus can slow the blood and oxygen supply to the baby by compressing the inferior vena cava, which brings the blood back to the heart after it circulates through the body. Change positions frequently. This may speed the progress of dilation, help morale, prevent stiffness, and increase comfort.

The most discouraging aspect of a plateau is that although the contractions are strong and you must work hard with them, you see no progress. In fact, frequently the contractions appear to grow stronger and stronger. You may be dilated 3 to 4 cm and be experiencing double-peak contractions similar to those described for transition. You may also feel nauseous, restless, fatigued, and irritable. Of course, you may not recognize these as symptoms of transition, as you are only dilated to 3 cm. The tendency at this time is to *panic*. "If this is early labor, I can't possibly cope with transition. *Help!*"

Labor partners need to keep alert to the different signs of progress. The degree of cervical dilation is not as accurate a guide as the intensity of the contractions and other symptoms the mother may experience. Keep in mind the physical and emotional signs of progress in labor (see pages 74–75), and do not hesitate to tell the mother of your observations. Once the mother experiences symptoms of transition, she is in transition, regardless of how far she is dilated. All at once, the dilation will catch up to the quality of the contractions the mother is having, and labor will progress rapidly.

As the labor partner, you should do all you can to support the mother. She can be very susceptible to vocal inflections and words. If you have a positive outlook and offer encouragement, she will feel positive. Remind her of her progress in other areas by telling her how the contractions may be producing effacement, descent, or a more favorable position of the baby for birth. Encourage her to urinate frequently and to change her position. Provide comfort measures for a backache if she has one. Use your love and support to keep her from becoming depressed or anxious.

BREECH POSITION

Most babies assume a **head-down** or **vertex position** by the eighth month. Because of the location of the placenta, a short umbilical cord, the shape of your pelvis, or other unknown reasons, however, your baby may assume a **breech position** in the uterus, with his head at the fundus and either buttocks or feet presenting at the cervix (see Figure 4.3). About three percent of all babies assume this position. You may be informed of this during a prenatal exam. Some birth attendants try to turn the baby by externally maneuvering his head down toward the pelvis. Occasionally this works, but sometimes the baby resumes his breech position. The breech may not be discovered until labor, when the person examining you tells you of the "funny head" (really the baby's buttocks) felt through the cervix.

Labor involving a breech may be different from that involving a vertex position. A longer first stage is common with breech presentations, because the soft buttocks or feet do not put sufficient pressure on the cervix. However, some breech labors progress very rapidly.

You may also experience backache and a decreased urge to push. With the baby in this position, measures are always taken to insure that the outlet of the pelvis is large enough to accommodate the baby's head. Your physician may determine this with a vaginal exam, ultrasound, or X-ray pelvimetry. The bony structures of the mother's pelvis and the baby's head can be seen on an X-ray. The baby's position, size, and head dimensions can thus be measured in relation to the pelvic size and shape. If the pelvis is not large enough for the baby to come through the pelvis, a cesarean delivery will be performed.

Because some early studies showed increased risks for babies in a breech position who were born vaginally, some doctors choose to perform a cesarean birth regardless of the size of the pelvis. More recent studies have shown the risks to be smaller than previously thought. Consequently, there now seems to be a slight trend toward vaginal birth. Once the decision has been made to deliver a breech baby vaginally, the birth should be continued in a gentle but efficient manner. The baby's head may not have time to mold and adjust to the birth canal, and more anesthesia may be needed. An anesthesiologist is often present for this purpose. Forceps may be used to assist the birth of the head.

MEDICAL TECHNOLOGY

Childbirth is a natural process, but women experiencing childbirth today are often aided by modern technology. The birth process is the same as it always was, but the technology changes the experience. Today's technology is such that many mothers and babies who might have died or been injured during childbirth before now live full and happy lives. This is due to such advances

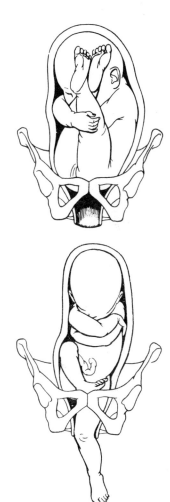

Figure 4.3
Breech Presentation
Sometimes, the baby assumes a buttocks-first or feet-first position.

as prenatal testing, induction or augmentation (stimulation) of labor, electronic fetal monitoring during labor, IVs, artificial rupture of the amniotic sac, and medication. Cesarean births and forceps are also examples of today's advanced medical procedures. Obviously, these procedures are not needed in every labor, but when necessary they can greatly enhance the outcome of childbirth.

Prenatal Testing

Tests may be done to determine how well the placenta is functioning and to assess the baby's maturity. Depending on the results of these tests, the pregnancy may be continued, labor may be initiated, or a cesarean birth may be planned. These tests include estriol level determination; the Oxytocin Challenge Test, or Stress Test (OCT); the Non-Stress Test (NST); amniocentesis; and ultrasound.

The **estriol determination test** shows how well the placenta is functioning. As the pregnancy advances, the placenta produces greater amounts of estriol, a form of estrogen. Estriol is found in the mother's blood and urine, and the amount can easily be determined. More than one test must be done to determine a trend. If there is a gradual or sudden drop in the estriol level, this may mean that the placenta is not functioning well. The decision to interrupt the pregnancy should not be based only on the estriol level. It is a safe and relatively inexpensive test, but it is not sufficiently accurate when used alone.

In the **Oxytocin Challenge Test (OCT)**, Pitocin, a synthetic form of the hormone oxytocin, is given to the mother intravenously to cause uterine contractions. An external monitor is used to assess the baby's response to these contractions.

First, a 20-minute reading of the baby's heartbeat is obtained to form the baseline (a recording of his heartbeat without contractions). Then the oxytocin is slowly administered until three contractions occur within ten minutes. The deviation of the baby's heartbeat from his normal pattern (baseline) in response to these contractions is evaluated. The test is considered "positive" if the fetal heart rate drops late in the contraction. This means that he may have trouble with labor, or that the placenta is no longer functioning properly. In this case, either an induction or cesarean birth may be planned. The problems with this test are (1) it must be done in the hospital,

(2) it places stress on the baby, (3) the Pitocin may start labor before the baby is ready, and (4) it is accurate only 75 percent of the time.

Many physicians are now using the **Non-Stress Test (NST)** before performing the OCT. An external monitor is again used to assess the baby's heart rate, but this time it evaluates the baby's response to his own movement. In a healthy baby, the heart rate increases when he moves. A "positive" test indicates fetal well-being. A baby who does not react to his own movement may have trouble in labor. If a nonreactive test is encountered (the heart rate does not increase when the baby moves), another NST may be done later, or an OCT may be performed.

The NST is inexpensive, may be done in a physician's office, does not place stress on the baby, and is a fairly accurate indicator of fetal well-being. The problem with this test is a lack of standardization; the range of normality is too wide and is subject to individual interpretation.

Another prenatal test is **amniocentesis**. In this test, amniotic fluid is withdrawn from the uterus. The fluid can then be tested for fetal abnormalities, antibody formation (Rh factor), and fetal maturity. Amniocentesis may also provide a means of treating the baby while he is still in the uterus (e.g., blood transfusions for blood incompatibility can be administered). Before amniocentesis, ultrasound is usually used to ascertain the baby's position and the placement of the placenta. Amniocentesis is not done routinely because of the possibility of bleeding, infection, premature labor, and injury to the baby.

The **ultrasound scan** directs sound waves toward the woman's abdomen and transmits an image of the baby and the placenta onto a screen. This is helpful in the detection of twins and in the confirmation of placenta previa (a condition in which the placenta is implanted in the lower uterus, partially or completely blocking the cervical opening).

Ultrasound may also be used to determine the due date by measuring the diameter of the baby's head. This is accurate to within one week before or one week after the estimated due date if done between the fourteenth and twentieth weeks of pregnancy. This information is valuable to the mother who may need to give birth early in order to have a healthy baby. Ultrasound may also be used to determine the growth rate of your baby. The safety of ultrasound has not been established, and the U.S. Food and Drug Administration has advised that it only be used when medically indicated. Parents should carefully weigh the information to be gained against any possible risks.

Labor Interventions

Induced or Augmented Labor

If tests indicate that labor should be medically initiated, the mother will be admitted to the birthing unit either the night before or the day on which the induction is scheduled. An IV drip is usually started in a vein in the lower arm or hand. After the needle is inserted, a tiny, flexible, plastic tube may be placed in the vein and the needle removed. The mother need not keep her arm still, and may continue to use effleurage.

The stimulation or induction of labor is usually accomplished by the administration of Pitocin through the IV drip. The frequency of the contractions is controlled by increasing or decreasing the rate of the flow of the IV fluid.

The interval between induced contractions is usually shorter than that between natural contractions. Usually, the contractions are regulated to come every three to four minutes. The character of induced contractions may differ slightly from natural ones. Induced contractions may appear to peak at the beginning rather than in the middle. This peak may drop off suddenly at the end of the contraction, or decrease gradually, beginning in the middle of the contraction. On the electronic fetal heart monitor tape, the contractions will not look different. The difference is in the mother's perception of the contraction.

Because of the rapid peak of the induced contraction, the mother must maintain her alertness and not be surprised by the contractions' intensity. It is extremely important to identify the character of the contractions and prepare for each one. It is often helpful to begin using the techniques several seconds before the contraction actually begins. Because these contractions are regular, the labor partner or nurse can use a watch to tell the mother when to start. Great determination and attention to techniques are required to effectively cope with induced labor. However, the stronger quality of the contractions produced by induction will often shorten labor.

Pitocin may also be used to stimulate or augment a labor that is already in progress, but has stopped or is not progressing well. Your birth attendant will decide whether to allow labor to progress at its own rate or to help it along. During one of your prenatal visits, discuss with your birth attendant his beliefs concerning labor augmentation.

Usually, once labor has been well established with the aid of Pitocin, the medication is

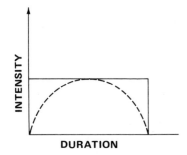

INTENSITY

DURATION

Figure 4.4
The Induced Labor
Contraction
These contractions are some-what different from natural con-tractions. Often intense in nature, the interval between contractions is quite short— usually only 3–4 minutes in length.

decreased or discontinued. The mother's body then continues the labor.

Because induced contractions are stronger, they may slow the blood flow through the placenta. The blood vessels that supply the placenta go through the muscle of the uterus. As the uterus forcefully contracts, these blood vessels are somewhat compressed. The baby is closely monitored to insure that he is receiving adequate oxygen through the placenta and is not being placed under stress by these contractions. Because of this increased risk, inductions for the convenience of the mother or doctor are infrequently performed, but when medically indicated, an induction can greatly increase the chance of a positive outcome.

Intravenous (IV) Fluids

During labor, an intravenous (IV) solution of sugar water is frequently administered. Many birth attendants believe that women should not eat or drink anything during labor. They worry that should an emergency occur and the mother require general anesthesia, she might vomit and aspirate the vomit into the lungs. In order to prevent dehydration, the birth attendant may order fluids to be given intravenously. The IV drip also allows access to a vein should medication be required.

Usually, a needle is inserted into the forearm and taped into place. Sometimes a thin plastic tube is inserted into the vein. When a catheter (a plastic tube) is used, the mother can freely move her arm.

Some birth attendants do not routinely use an IV drip during labor, but instead allow the mother to drink small quantities of fluid. They believe that should vomiting occur, the highly acidic gastric secretions would produce more problems than would any foods or fluids that the mother might have ingested. They also feel that restricting the mother's activities during labor may increase her discomfort.

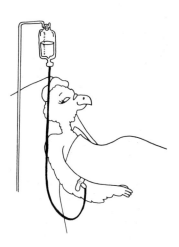

Fetal Monitoring

Your baby's reaction to labor will be monitored by observing any changes in his heart rate that occur in response to the uterine contractions. This can be done with a stethoscope or with the electronic fetal monitor (EFM), an ultrasound device.

The stethoscope has the advantage of not restricting the mother's movements during labor. Freedom of movement is important during labor, as it enables the mother to walk or to choose other positions that are comfortable for her. The disadvantage of using a stethoscope is that frequently the baby's heart rate cannot be heard during the contraction, and the attendant or nurse must assess his response between contractions when the uterine muscle is relaxed.

The EFM uses intermittent sound waves to detect and record the baby's heart rate. Unlike the stethoscope, it places limits on the mother's mobility. Its advantage is that it allows continous monitoring of the fetal heartbeat, even during contractions.

There are two types of electronic fetal monitors: the external monitor and the internal monitor. The external monitor consists of two disks that are placed on the mother's abdomen. One of these disks is placed at the fundus (the top portion of the uterus) to monitor the contractions, and the other is placed lower, to register the baby's heartbeat. This information is recorded on a graph similar to an electrocardiograph (EKG). You may not be able to perform effleurage easily when using the external monitor. Try to find a comfortable position before the monitor is applied. When you change positions, the placement of the monitors may need to be adjusted.

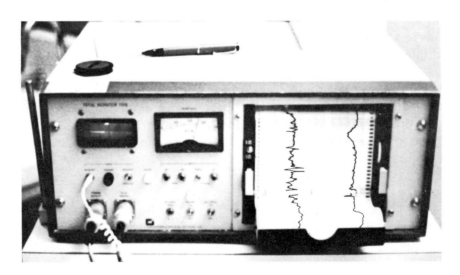

Figure 4.5
The Electronic Fetal Monitor
The EFM records and prints out graphs of uterine contractions and fetal heartbeats.

The internal monitor consists of two probes that are inserted through the vagina and into the opening in the cervix. One is a tube filled with water. This tube records the intensity of the uterine contractions. The other probe is attached to the baby's head and records his heartbeat.

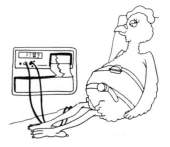

The bag of waters must be broken for internal monitoring. If the amniotic sac does not break on its own, the birth attendant may break it. To do this, he inserts two fingers into the vagina and touches the bag of waters (the amniotic sac), which can be felt bulging through the cervical opening. He then guides an amnihook along his fingers and makes a small nick in the amniotic sac. The amnihook looks like a flat crochet hook with a small sharp hook at the end. Except for the discomfort you may feel during the pelvic examination, this procedure is painless.

Labor may be shortened somewhat by breaking the bag of waters. The uterus can contract more forcefully, since the amount of fluid within the uterus is decreased. Although rupturing the membranes shortens labor, some birth attendants are concerned about the greater stress that may be placed on the baby due to the absence of the cushion of amniotic fluid. Another problem is that once the bag of waters is broken, the sterile environment of the baby is no longer intact. This "sets the clock ticking," providing a limited range of time in which the baby must be born to avoid increased chances of infection.

The bottom line of the monitor tape (see Figure 4.6, page 104) shows the uterine contractions. They are coming every 3 minutes, and lasting approximately 60 seconds. Each vertical line on this tape represents 60 seconds. Your own monitor may be adjusted to show more or less time between the vertical lines.

The monitors are used primarily to observe closely the baby's reaction to the contractions, and to detect any abnormal patterns. In the illustration, the baby's heart rate is good, as is indicated by the very jagged line (called variability). The more jagged the line, the better the heartbeat. Sometimes the heart rate drops or increases sharply, but immediately returns to the normal range. This is a normal pattern. An abnormal one occurs when the heart rate drops and slowly returns to normal, forming a "U" or "V" shape. A single rise or dip in the baby's heart rate is not significant, but if it happens repeatedly, the cause must be determined and appropriate measures initiated.

Often, just changing the mother's position can release the pressure on the baby or the umbilical cord and relieve the strain on the baby, thus returning his heart rate to normal. At other times, the situation can only be remedied by the birth of the baby. In this case, a forceps delivery would be performed if birth were imminent, and a cesarean delivery would be performed if dilation were not complete.

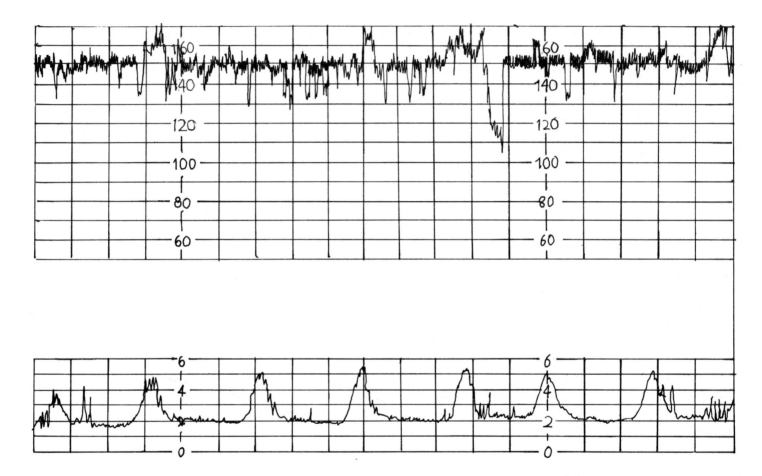

Figure 4.6
The Electronic
Fetal Monitor Readout
The top line represents the
baby's heartbeat. The bottom
line represents the uterine contractions.

Because not all heart rate patterns that appear abnormal mean that the baby is under stress, many birth attendants now use the monitor tracing in conjunction with the fetal scalp pH test. In this test, a drop of the baby's blood is analyzed to determine if he really is in distress before any decision is made to intervene.

The routine use of monitors has been questioned. Studies have been cited showing inaccurate recordings of fetal distress based on printouts that are subject to interpretation. The routine use of monitors may be responsible for some unnecessary cesarean births. There is also the possibility that because of maternal immobility ("Don't change position because we can't get a good reading of the baby's heartbeat when you do"), other situations arise requiring intervention. For example, the mother may be uncomfortable in one position and thus take medication for pain relief. Medication frequently slows labor, requiring measures to stimulate or augment the contractions. (See page 100.)

Some couples like the EFM because it allows them to accurately determine when the contractions are beginning, often before they can be felt by the mother. She may benefit from this advance warning by being able to begin her techniques before the contraction starts. Couples may also feel reassured by being able to see the baby's heartbeat continuously, and by the fact that the EFM enables problems to be detected while they can still be corrected.

Other couples do not like the monitors because of the decreased freedom and the "unnaturalness" of the machines. Some have felt that more attention was paid to the machine than to the mother, and have resented how impersonal the technology has made their birth experience.

Research done on the subject of the routine use of EFM shows conflicting results. Some studies indicate benefits, and other studies indicate no benefits. As with other ultrasound devices, research has not proven the existence of either long-term benefits or long-term hazards. You should discuss your concerns about electronic fetal heart monitoring with your birth attendant prior to your labor.

Medications for Labor and Birth

It is essential to discuss with your birth attendant his feelings about the use of medication and anesthesia during labor. Let him know what your desires are, and try to reach an agreement. You should do this before labor, so that you will not be surprised during labor. The following is a chart of the commonly used analgesics and anesthetics, their desired effects, and their unwanted effects. See page 5 for a discussion of the role of medication in labor and birth.

LABOR AND BIRTH MEDICATIONS

Type	Name	Administration	Possible Effects on Mother	Possible Effects on Baby
Analgesics Used to reduce or abolish pain or to alter perception of pain without loss of consciousness.	Demerol	Given IM or IV. Lasts 2–3 hours.	Hypotension (decreased blood pressure), euphoria, dizziness, dry mouth, decreased respiration, nausea, vomiting, and tremors. May decrease uterine contractions.	If given within 1 hour of birth, no apparent side effects. If given between 1 and 3 hours before birth, baby may have respiratory depression. Behavior may be altered for several days.
	Nisentil	Given subcutaneously or IV. Lasts 1½–2 hours.	Euphoria or depression, sedation, dizziness, sweating, nausea, and respiratory distress.	Depression.
Tranquilizers Used to relieve tension and anxiety, these drugs produce a state of mental tranquility without drowsiness. They are frequently used with narcotics to enhance the narcotic action while decreasing the required dosage.	Vistaril	Given IM or IV. Lasts 3–4 hours.	Drowsiness, dizziness, and dry mouth.	Unknown.
	Valium	Given IM or IV. Lasts 3–4 hours.	Drowsiness, confusion, hypotension, and retention of urine.	Produces beat-to-beat variations in baby's heart tones, decreased muscle tone, hypothermia, and decreased attentiveness.
	Phenergan	Given IM or IV. Lasts 6–8 hours.	Prevents nausea and vomiting. May produce drowsiness, central nervous system depression, confusion, and hypotension.	Unknown.
	Largon	Given IM or IV. Lasts about 3 hours.	Dry mouth, increased blood pressure, drowsiness, dizziness, and central nervous system depression.	Unknown.

LABOR AND BIRTH MEDICATIONS—*Continued*

Type	Name	Administration	Possible Effects on Mother	Possible Effects on Baby
Anesthetics				
Used to completely block pain impulses to the brain, thus causing total loss of sensation. Depending on site chosen, the anesthesia will numb either a local or a more general area.	Paracervical Block	Injected on each side of the cervix, from 3 cm to complete dilation. Blocks uterine pain. Lasts from 45 minutes to 2 hours.	None if proper dosage and techniques are used. May slow contractions.	Decreased heart rate in 2%–70%, depending on dosage and drug used. Most danger occurs if baby is born during fetal heart rate depression. Injury to baby possible during administration.
	Pudendal Block	Injected into each pudendal nerve at the level of the ischial spines. For birth and episiotomy repair only.	Loss of bearing-down reflex if done properly. Some pain during administration.	Once in mother's bloodstream, quickly crosses placenta and may depress fetal respiration.
	Caudal Epidural	Injected into caudal canal below spinal cord after 5 cm dilation. Dose may be repeated. For labor, birth, and episiotomy repair.	May prolong labor. Hypotension, hypertension, or hypoventilation. Decreased muscle tone. Loss of bearing-down reflex with need for forceps. 5% failure rate.	Subtle neonatal changes, behavior alterations, and decreased muscle tone.
	Lumbar Epidural	Injected into space around spinal cord, at 6–7 cm dilation. May be repeated. Complete pain relief for labor, birth, and episiotomy repair. Technically difficult. May be used for cesarean birth.	Hypotension, depression. May decrease uterine contractions for 10–30 minutes. Loss of bearing-down reflex. Forceps may be needed. 3% failure rate.	Subtle neonatal changes, behavior alterations, and decreased muscle tone.

LABOR AND BIRTH MEDICATIONS—*Continued*

Type	Name	Administration	Possible Effects on Mother	Possible Effects on Baby
Analgesics	Spinal	Injected into spinal fluid. For cesareans or other operative births. Lasts 1–3 hours.	For cesarean, numbs from below navel to toes. Hypotension and headaches may result. Reduced bladder control is common. Loss of urge to push.	Oxygen deprivation due to hypotension in mother.
	Saddle Block	Injected into spinal fluid. Lasts 1½–3 hours.	Numbs perineum and inner thighs. Feet can sense, but not move. Loss of urge to push. Forceps necessary.	Same as spinal.
	General	Inhaled through mask. Complete pain relief; loss of consciousness. For emergency cesareans or other operative births.	Nausea and vomiting. Deep anesthesia depresses central nervous system, cardiac system, and respiratory system.	Crosses placenta easily; deep anesthesia effects same as for mother.
	Local	Injected into perineum. For repair of episiotomy only.	May not take effect.	Decreased muscle tone.

Birth Interventions

Cesarean Birth

A cesarean delivery is performed when a vaginal birth is impossible or inadvisable.

One reason for performing a cesarean birth is cephalopelvic disproportion, a condition in which the baby's head is too large to fit through the mother's pelvis. Another reason is a previous cesarean birth; in this case, most physicians elect to do a repeat cesarean. Fresh bleeding during labor may indicate that the placenta is abnormally situated (placenta previa) or that it has begun to prematurely separate (abruptio placentae). In these cases, a vaginal birth may compromise the health or life of both mother and baby. Another indication for surgery is that either mother or baby exhibits distress.

A cesarean birth is performed either in a surgical area or in a delivery room that has been set up for that purpose. If you are to have a cesarean birth, do not be alarmed at the number of people present. The birth team usually consists of the doctor, his assistant, an anesthetist, two nurses, and a pediatrician. The mother receives additional preparation for the birth. The abdominal and pubic hair may be shaved. A catheter is usually inserted into the bladder to remove the urine until the mother has recovered from the anesthesia. An IV drip is started to provide the mother with sugar and water both during the surgery and afterwards. After surgery, the mother gradually begins eating, first liquids, then solids. Until that time, she receives nourishment from the IV. The IV also provides the birth attendant with easy access to a vein should an emergency arise and medication, blood, or fluid need to be administered quickly.

Usually the mother lies on her back, with a pillow tilting her slightly to the left. A ground plate to prevent electric shock is placed under her, because electrocautery may be used during the surgery to close blood vessels. An electrocardiograph may also be used during surgery to monitor the mother's heart rate. The mother's abdomen is washed with an antiseptic, and then covered with sterile towels so that only the incision site is exposed. An "anesthesic" or "surgical" drape is placed over a metal frame around the mother's chest. This keeps the mother from actually seeing the incision and birth, and prevents contamination from coughing or sneezing.

The anesthesia used depends on the preferences of the mother and doctor and the reason for the cesarean. If this is an emergency procedure due to fetal or maternal distress, the anesthesia of choice will probably be general anesthesia, because it can be rapidly administered. If there is more time, the mother or doctor may opt for an epidural or spinal anesthetic. This allows the mother to remain awake, but anesthetizes her from her navel to her toes. Because of the drape between her face and abdomen, she cannot actually see the baby being born. However, the anesthetist often informs her of what is happening, and she can see and hear her infant as soon as he is born.

In many hospitals, the partner is allowed to be present for the birth. He can then provide emotional support for the mother and share in the birth of the child. Neither the mother nor the coach can see the surgery unless they look in a mirror that may be placed above the table for their viewing, or the partner looks over the drape. Some hospitals prefer that the partner take a cesarean childbirth class if he is to be present at the cesarean birth. Check the policies in your area if a cesarean birth is a possibility.

The abdominal incision may be either vertical (from the navel downward) or horizontal (just within the area of the pubic hair—called a "bikini cut" because you can wear a skimpy one later without a scar showing).

After the abdominal incision is made, an incision is made into the uterus. This, also, can be either vertical or horizontal. Usually the uterine incision is made horizontally in a semicircular fashion in the lower part of the uterus, above the cervix. This area of the muscle does not contract during labor, so there is less danger of the scar breaking open during subsequent labors. The vertical uterine incision, called the "classical" incision, is not often used today unless the baby is very large, or the placenta is lying low in the uterus.

The doctor may use forceps (see page 113), a vacuum extractor (see page 114), or his hands to lift the baby out of the uterus. The baby may have a lot of mucus in his mouth and upper chest area, because it has not been rhythmically massaged out as it would have been in a vaginal birth. The birth attendant suctions out this mucus. When a cesarean is performed because of a prolonged labor without progress, the baby's head may be molded. Otherwise the baby's head is rounded. The baby is held up for the mother to see, and is then given to the mother to hold, placed in a warmer in the birth area, or taken to the nursery. What happens following the birth depends on the baby's response to birth. After an emergency cesarean birth, the baby is usually taken to the nursery for observation.

Meanwhile, the doctor suctions out the amniotic fluid and lifts out the placenta. He repairs the incision, beginning with the uterus. The individual muscle layers of the abdomen are then

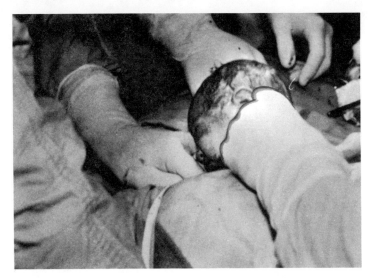

In a cesarean birth, the baby is lifted out of the uterus. Here, the baby's head is just beginning to emerge through the incision.

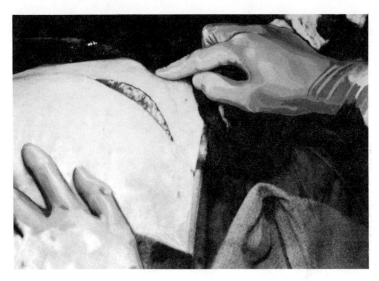

After the placenta is removed and the uterine incision is closed, the abdominal incision is repaired.

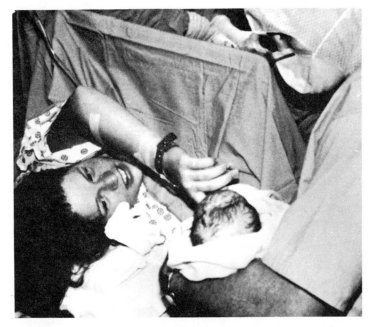

After birth, the proud parents examine their newborn child.

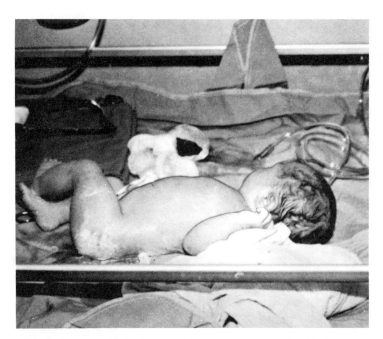

Sometimes, the baby is placed in a warmer soon after birth.

closed. Finally, the doctor closes the abdominal incision with stitches, clamps, or surgical tape. The entire procedure takes about one hour. In an emergency, the baby can be born within 5 minutes, but it takes about 45 minutes to repair the incision, because each layer of muscle or skin is repaired individually.

After birth, the mother's vital signs (pulse and blood pressure) are monitored. The nurse manually checks the uterus to make sure it is contracting to prevent excessive bleeding. If it is not contracting, she may need to massage the uterus. This can be very uncomfortable, and may require conscious relaxation and breathing techniques if the anesthesia is wearing off. It is most commonly done in the recovery area.

When the mother recovers from the anesthesia, she is usually taken to a postpartum room. A major discomfort following a cesarean is intestinal gas. The sooner the new mother gets up and walks around, the faster she will recover and the less gas she will have. Although the idea of getting up and walking may seem impossible (she will need help at first), it will make her feel better. She will feel even better if she stands and walks tall, rather than slumping over to protect her very sore abdomen. Just as contracting the pelvic floor helps heal an episiotomy, contracting the abdominal muscles, although painful, helps heal an abdominal incision. Breathing techniques may aid in alleviating the discomfort.

Because a cesarean birth requires abdominal surgery, the mother usually stays in the hospital for five to seven days. Most prepared women who require a cesarean birth enjoy very rapid recoveries. This is probably due to the fact that the prepared mother experiences less tension and fear than does one who lacks preparation.

It is becoming increasingly common for women who had previous cesarean births to give birth vaginally. The rule "once a cesarean, always a cesarean" is changing as new techniques are developed for use during cesarean births. As long as the cause for the cesarean is not a recurring one, such as a small pelvis, there is a good chance that the woman can give birth vaginally. The type of incision, too, must be considered when determining if a conventional delivery is possible. A horizontal incision that was made just above the cervix, in an area that does not contract during labor, favors vaginal delivery. Other factors that favor vaginal birth include a vertex presentation with head well down in the birth canal at the beginning of labor, a soft stretchy cervix, and a baby that is not exceptionally large. The nutritional and health status of the mother during her pregnancy is also considered. Facilities for continuous fetal monitoring during labor should be available, as well as a delivery room and a surgical staff, should an emergency arise.

An anesthesiologist and pediatrician should be on call.

The incidence of cesarean births in the United States averages about 15 percent (lower in some areas and higher in others). Some of these are planned cesareans, but many are not. A cesarean is "unplanned" when the mother does not know prior to going into labor that she will have a cesarean birth. No matter what the cause, many women feel guilty or disappointed after a cesarean birth. They may feel that their bodies have failed them, or that if they had just practiced relaxation longer they could have given birth vaginally. In most cases the situation was unavoidable, and the mother could not have done anything to change the outcome. She is not a failure! She is a mother whose baby was born via an abdominal rather than a vaginal route. The door was closed, so a window was used. In many areas of the country there are support groups that provide cesarean information and help mothers who have had cesarean births. If you want more information about these groups, contact your doctor, hospital, or childbirth education group.

Forceps and Vacuum Extraction

Forceps look like metal salad tongs and function like a pair of hands. They are used to turn the baby into a better position for birth, or to assist the baby down the birth canal.

There are several circumstances that may require the use of forceps. First, a slight disproportion may exist between the size of the baby and the birth canal (cephalopelvic disproportion). Second, after pushing for a long time, both the uterus and mother may become fatigued, and the mother's pushing efforts may consequently be ineffective. Third, the baby's heart rate may show that he is tired, thus indicating the need for a rapid delivery. Fourth, a breech presentation, which sometimes prevents the head from molding as it descends through the birth canal, may require the aid of forceps to deliver the baby's head. Fifth, the baby in a posterior presentation, who has the back of his head lying against his mother's back, may need assistance. As he descends through the vagina, his head tends to bend backwards, pushing him against the rectum instead of down the birth canal. In this case, forceps may be used to turn the baby's head, thus facilitating his birth. Forceps may also be indicated if the mother has had spinal, caudal, or epidural anesthesia, any of which may eliminate her urge to bear down and cause a relaxation of the muscles that produce the bearing-down effort.

The application of forceps may be low, mid, or high. Low forceps are used when the baby is

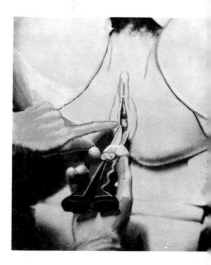

Figure 4.7
Forceps Delivery.
Forceps may be used to correct the baby's position or to assist the baby down the birth canal.

situated low in the vagina and needs only a little assistance to be born. The forceps are lubricated with warm sterile water and gently applied to both sides of his head. Used during a contraction, so that all forces are working together—the uterus, the mother, and the birth attendant—forceps assist the baby's head through the vaginal opening. When his head is almost out, the forceps are removed. The rest of the baby is born as usual.

Mid forceps are used when the baby is halfway up the vagina. High forceps are used when the baby is still within the uterus. Because of the danger associated with the use of high forceps, most physicians elect to do a cesarean birth instead of high forceps. There is excessive pressure exerted on the baby during a high-forceps-assisted birth.

Infants occasionally have slight, superficial bruises from the forceps. These are due to the breaking of fragile capillaries during birth, and disappear within a few days. They do not indicate problems for the baby.

Vacuum extraction is an option in some areas of the country. This procedure uses suction instead of forceps. A small suction cup is placed on the baby's head, and the suction, which can be adjusted by the physician, helps to ease the baby out through the birth canal. The baby's head will have slight swelling where the suction cup was placed, but this is temporary.

THE PARTNER'S ROLE IN NONCONFORMING LABORS

Perhaps the single most important factor affecting a woman's response to labor is the quality of assistance she receives from her labor partner. Unpleasant situations may occur during labor, but the mother's response to them can be greatly improved by her partner's support.
by her partner's support.

Back labor is an example of one unavoidable situation that can be made more bearable by the partner. Depression caused by a lack of progress during a plateau also can be decreased by loving support. Fear of the intensity of future contractions can be reduced or eliminated by informing the mother of the progress of labor. The positive effect that good labor support has on the mother cannot be overemphasized.

Here are some suggestions that may aid you in coping with labor. While these guidelines will be helpful during any labor, they will be of particular value during a nonconforming labor, when the demands on both the mother and the labor partner are the greatest.

- Bring a sandwich and something to drink for yourself so that you will not have to leave the labor room if you get hungry or thirsty.
- If the mother needs support for her lower back during labor, ask for an extra pillow to place under her back (a rolled blanket or sheet will do). You can also elevate the head and knee portion of the bed to make her more comfortable.
- Keep your fingertips or palms lightly above the mother's navel so you can feel the uterine muscle tighten before she feels any sensation from it. Announce "contraction is beginning" and call "15 seconds . . . 30 seconds . . . 45 seconds . . . , etc." until the muscle starts to relax again. In transition, vary the count of the seconds: "29 . . . 44 . . . 64 . . . , etc." This may provide a welcome change of pace.
- Be firm and consistent in telling her to relax and to conserve her energy for the work yet to come. Stroke constantly during contractions unless applying back pressure. Lovingly and firmly keep her attention focused on her work.
- Be armed with moral support and add continuous encouragement and praise no matter how long the labor may be. Remain calm.
- Even if you feel discouraged or doubtful, try to keep those feelings to yourself. A woman in labor can be supersensitive to the attitudes and reactions of those around her. If you give up, she may too.
- After the membranes rupture, the contractions almost always become stronger. Remind the mother of this and suggest a change in the breathing technique if necessary. If her control is threatened by a very strong contraction, keep her breathing and concentrating until it is over. It may help to lean close to her and breathe with her or forcefully tell her how to breathe. Eye contact during these contractions is very helpful.
- Sponge her face with a washcloth and ice water if she feels drowsy or uncomfortably warm. The feeling that she would rather go to sleep and forget about the entire thing is very common during labor. The body must be at rest, but not the mind. If the mind is not kept alert, the pain threshold is greatly reduced. Help her to analyze the character of her contractions to determine the appropriate response.
- A change in the mother's position is often a good idea, especially when the labor is long. Pillows placed under her arms, head, and knees, or a change in the position of the bed will often make her more comfortable. The labor position should be changed more frequently if she has back labor, unless otherwise directed by the doctor or staff.

- In the event of backache, apply firm pressure to counteract the feeling during a contraction. It will probably be felt very low in the sacrum, or the small of the back. Use lotion or powder to avoid irritating the skin while applying pressure. An ice bag applied to the mother's back may also help this discomfort, as will massage or pressure from tennis balls or containers filled with ice. The thumb-pressure massage (Shiatsu) and the passive pelvic rock are very helpful during back labor.

- Remind the mother to try to urinate every hour to prevent unnecessary discomfort from a full bladder.

- Apply lip balm to her lips, powder her abdomen, offer her gum or sour lollipops to moisten her dry mouth, give her ice chips to suck on if the doctor has given his permission, and hang up the object that you have brought for her to focus on.

- Write down the duration and type of contractions the mother is having, the breathing she is doing, her progress in effacement and dilation, and any other significant things that occur. You will probably not remember these things, and may want this information in the future, as it will be helpful when you both write your labor reports.

- Suggest a change in breathing techniques if the one being used is no longer effective. Habit is easily acquired, and because the mother is so busy concentrating, she may forget to change her breathing.

- Between 7 and 10 cm dilation, the contractions are at their strongest. Remind her that this is the most difficult period, but also the shortest. The contractions will not get any harder than they are now. During transition, she may feel panicky and snap back at you, so be prepared, and do not take offense. Remind her that the birth of your baby is now very near! Do not be frightened by the way she reacts during the transition phase. These are strong contractions, but you must go on; she needs your strength. She may say, "I can't do it," and you may wonder what you can do to help. You may be concerned by the intensity of the contractions and by her responses. Encourage her, be strong, and give her your strength. Review all of the relaxation techniques, breathing techniques, and comfort measures. Use every trick in the book to reinforce the skills you have learned. If necessary, do the effleurage for her if she is unable to. The pressure of the massage required may increase or decrease during transition. Between contractions, ask the mother which she prefers.

● Remind her to push properly, should she forget. Make sure she does not strain her neck instead of her abdominal muscles, and keep reminding her to relax her lips and perineum. Help support her shoulders and neck while pushing. Do this by putting your arms under the pillow. Do not lift her up. Allow her to find the position that is most comfortable for her; then support her in that position. Remind her to allow the contraction to build up before she begins pushing. Pushing too soon with a contraction is both useless and exhausting.

Throughout this manual, we have explained what you should do during practice and labor. You may still have some reservations about the entire process and your role in it. Perhaps you think that you are wasting your time, that the method is not sufficiently effective, or that the mother is not sufficiently strong. We understand these feelings, because many people in our classes felt that way before labor. It may encourage you to know that they didn't feel that way after they went through labor.

Many couples have been pleasantly surprised by how the techniques helped them during labor. Both fathers and mothers discovered strengths they didn't realize they possessed, and entered parenthood feeling able and eager to cope with the stress of raising the child they had worked so hard to have.

Chapter Five
Your New Family: Infant Care and Postpartum Adjustment

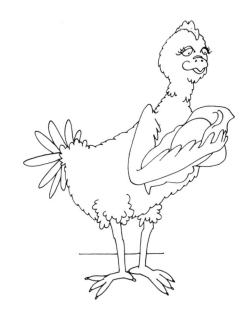

EARLY POSTPARTUM INFANT CARE

After birth, your baby's main needs will be for air and warmth. The nursing staff will suction mucus out of his nose and mouth to facilitate his breathing. Your baby will also be kept warm for several hours after birth while he adjusts to the temperature outside the uterus. This is done by allowing you to hold him next to your body, by wrapping him in extra blankets, or by placing him in a heated crib. At first he will simply be dried off and wrapped in a blanket. Later he will be bathed to wash off any amniotic fluid, vernix, or blood that may be left from the passage down the birth canal.

State law requires that drops or ointment be placed into the baby's eyes to prevent blindness (gonorrheal conjunctivitis) caused by venereal disease. Usually, silver nitrate is used for this purpose. However, as silver nitrate will irritate his eyes, try to see if this can be postponed for a couple hours, or suggest that nonirritating erythromycin or tetracycline ointment be used so that you will have a chance to get acquainted with him. Your baby can see from the moment of birth, but he has a fixed point of focus that is about eight to nine inches.

At some point, your baby will be weighed and measured. The doctor will also give him a complete physical examination, and will share his findings with you. The baby's urine and blood will be tested. Since a newborn cannot produce his own Vitamin K, your baby may be given a Vitamin K injection to lessen the chance of bleeding from the umbilical cord or circumcision.

Because he continuously received nutrients from the placenta before birth, your baby may not be hungry for a while. Some babies nurse immediately after birth, and therefore receive some nutrients from the colostrum (an early form of breast milk). More often, however, this is a time of exploration. The baby will seriously nurse later. A bottle-fed baby is given sugar water a few hours after birth. Most of the baby's time immediately after birth should be spent resting and getting acquainted with his new environment and his family.

Circumcision

If your baby is a boy, the question of circumcision will come up. This procedure of cutting off the foreskin of the penis has been performed extensively in the United States during the last 75 to 100 years. Many other countries do not do this routinely. There is considerable discussion today as to whether the procedure is necessary. Many feel that it should not be done. An ad hoc committee of the American Academy of Pediatrics suggested that the procedure not be done because of the possibility of complications, the pain the baby experiences, and the lack of proof of any possible benefit.

Many couples still prefer to have their babies circumcised. They believe that it is easier to clean the penis if the foreskin is gone, that their child will be considered different and become sexually maladjusted if he is not circumcised, and that it will save the boy from future surgery. None of these theories appears to be substantiated by research findings. Cleaning the penis is slightly different, but not harder, in an uncircumcised male. The foreskin should be gently slid back only as far as it can easily go to expose the head of the penis while bathing. Do not forcibly retract the foreskin; it usually retracts completely by the time the child is five years old. Sexual maladjustment does not appear to occur. Apparently few boys or men look at each other closely enough in locker rooms to notice who is circumcised and who is not; if they do notice, they do not appear to care. Increased sensations during intercourse have been reported by those who are uncircumcised. The incidence of circumcision done in later years is difficult to determine, as it may be done on an outpatient basis. The procedure is done with local anesthesia (none is routinely given to the newborn), and recovery is fairly rapid.

This is another procedure that parents should discuss together and with their baby's physician before labor begins. It will be difficult to make an informed decision on this matter once you are in the hospital.

Bonding and Rooming-In

The first couple of hours of a baby's life can be very precious. You will have waited so long for this moment, and will be eager to begin a loving relationship through a natural process called **bonding**. Your new baby will be marvelously equipped to help you fall in love with him. He will be alert and responsive, and will look intently into your eyes. As you gaze into his eyes, you will be charmed by his innocence and helplessness.

Besides looking at you intently, your baby will also listen to you intently. If he is restless, just talking to him may quiet him. How powerful and loving you will feel when he so readily responds to your voice! Fathers, not just mothers, notice this response. This will be especially true if the father talked to his baby when it was in the uterus. (It may seem strange to visualize the father bending down over a big tummy and talking to it, but many fathers feel that this is one way in which they can get to know their baby before it is born.) Your baby will not just look at and listen to you, but will cuddle into your body as you hold him. You will want to keep on holding his small, warm, cuddly body forever! Is this love?

Usually, your baby will spend his first couple of hours with you. Depending on his condition and the arrangements you have made with your birth attendant, the baby will then either stay with your or go to a nursery. Many birthing areas now offer **rooming-in**, an arrangement that allows the baby to stay with his mother in her room for specific periods of time. With full rooming-in, the baby stays with the mother 24 hours a day until she goes home. With flexible rooming-in, the baby stays with the mother most of the time, but goes to a nursery when the mother sleeps, showers, or has visitors.

Rooming-in has some definite advantages. If this is your first baby, you will get an opportunity to care for him and ask questions of the nurses before you go home. When you are on your own at home you will feel more confident in your ability to care for your baby. If this is your second baby, this will be a good time to get acquainted with him—just the two of you alone. Once you

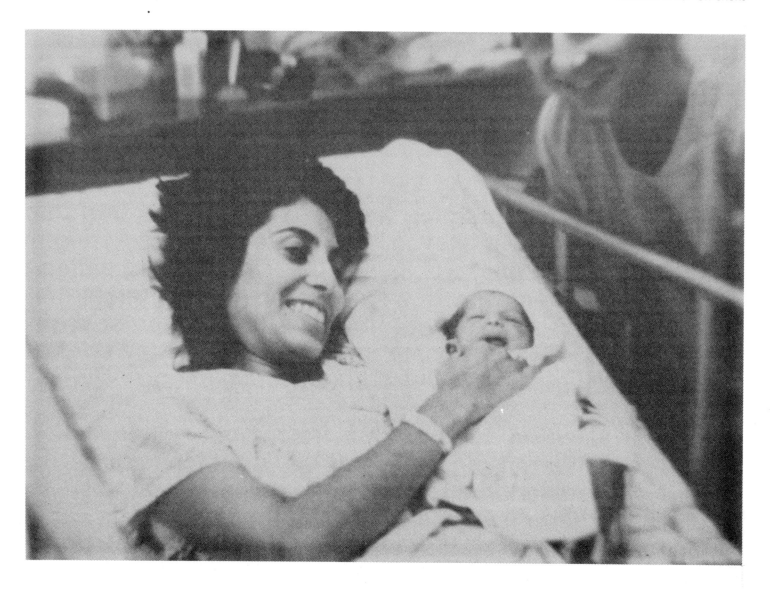

get home, there will be others sharing your attention. This is even more significant if you have several children at home. Breastfeeding, also, is more easily established with rooming-in.

Many women rest better when their babies are with them than they do when they have to wonder what is happening to their child and have to travel to a central nursery to find out. Some women become tense and restless when they are separated from their newborns. *In utero*, the baby usually sleeps when the mother does (that is, once he gets settled down). If you have full rooming-in, and your baby sleeps in your room at night, you will still essentially be on the same schedule. Sometimes the bright lights, noise, and activity of a central nursery disrupt the baby's schedule.

Some women prefer not to have their baby room in with them. They enjoy the freedom from responsibility, and the freedom to do what they want (within limits, of course) for a time before going home. Others believe that they rest better when they have someone else care for their baby. The subject of rooming-in, and the various types of rooming-in arrangements, should be discussed with your birth attendant.

The first days of your new baby's life may be some of the best days of your life. Pregnancy will be over, and you will probably be glad of that. You will be in awe of what you have done. You will be aware of your need for rest, and should try to get as much as possible. While you are in bed resting, read the next section of this book to prepare yourself for the next few weeks, which may *not* be the best weeks of your life.

THE FIRST WEEKS AT HOME

It would be unfair to end this manual with the baby's birth and not prepare you in some way for what happens afterwards. Birth is not only an end to pregnancy. It is the beginning of a new life—not just for the baby, but for the parents also. Your life will *never* be the same again, and this does take some adjustment. Your active participation in the birth of your baby may make this adjustment easier, but it is never really easy for anyone.

You are probably looking forward to your child's birth, and may believe that you will have no trouble adjusting to your new situation. After all, pregnancy has not changed you much, and you plan to take parenthood in stride also. We understand that now you may not accept the contents of this chapter. Put this book in a place where you will be able to find it easily after the birth of your child. To some degree, everyone experiences the feelings described here, and you may find solace in reading this later.

Physical and Emotional Adjustments

Your child will be a source of great happiness. At times you will feel such strong, intense love that you may feel like bursting with joy. You will sit and look at your sleeping angel and think that there is nothing better in the world than being the parent of your baby. When he is awake you will be fascinated by the many things he does. Babies have the most flexible facial muscles, and the faces they make are of endless variety. Babies seem to always be in motion, either moving their arms or legs or both. There is no denying the fact that parenthood is delightful. But you may also experience negative emotions toward both your child and your life after his birth. In the following section we will discuss some of these negative feelings—not because they are the most common of all feelings, but because they are so distressing.

One of these first feelings may be a lack of affection for your baby. The mother most often notices this. She has become accustomed to experiencing her child within her, and now must adjust to the fact that her baby is a separate person. Many parents expect to feel an immediate surge of love for their newborn, and are concerned when they do not feel this way. Do not worry. There is usually a period of time from several hours to several weeks before the parents grow to love their child.

After you have had your baby home for a few days, you may find that you are not well prepared for parenthood. Some mothers who used Lamaze for the birth of their children feel like super-women. They gave birth with confidence and felt wonderful and full of energy in the hospital. After birth, however, they are confronted with their new babies, and do not understand why they do not feel like superwomen anymore.

Contrary to some popularly held beliefs, there is no instinct that tells parents how to hold, change, diaper, or feed their children. These are all learned skills. Through playing with dolls in childhood, many women gained some idea of how these tasks should be done, but a living, squirming baby is very different from a lifeless doll. Further, many men and women have never held a small infant or even seen another person care for a new baby. Most mothers and fathers enter parenthood without knowing anything about the daily tasks of caring for their children, except for what they have read. Suddenly, the baby is there! Now what? This may produce anxiety, especially for the mother, because she feels that she should know what to do. Often the father also feels that his wife should know, and offers her no support during this trying period.

Most women feel somewhat inadequate, but hide their feelings and pretend that they have everything under control. This only serves to perpetuate the myth of a "maternal instinct" and prevent the mother from getting the help that might be forthcoming if she admitted her feelings to someone she trusts. Some parents go to the other extreme and express their feelings of inadequacy to everyone, getting help and advice from all sources. They are then in a quandary, because they do not know whom to believe. If this is not their first child, the parents get less help because everyone expects them to know everything already. But no child is like his sibling, and even if you have other children you may encounter feelings of inadequacy.

Some feelings of inadequacy can be eliminated by remembering that you were mothering your baby long before birth. You soothed him when he was fussy or uncomfortable. When your baby was active, what kind of things did you do? Talk to him? Massage him through your abdomen? Rock him by walking? Sing to him? The things you did before birth will also help soothe him after he is born.

You must use your common sense when raising children. You have probably seen a new baby in 90 degree weather dressed in a sweater, booties, hat, and blankets. The baby was fussy, and the parents did not know what was wrong, because he had just eaten and was dry. What would bother you will probably also annoy your baby. When the baby cries, check first to see if he is hungry, hot or cold, bothered by noise, frustrated (wants to roll over but cannot yet), tired, or bored. Unless he has a diaper rash, a new baby will probably not be bothered by warm, moist diapers. There are other causes of crying, but these are some of the most common. Another frequent cause of crying is the need to be held and loved. Different babies require different amounts of attention, and each has his own personality at birth. Sometimes you can guess what your child will be like by his activity level in the uterus. Active children may need more attention than quiet children. Observe how much attention your baby needs before he is soothed.

Some babies soothe themselves after a couple minutes of crying, while others stop crying as soon as they see your face or hear your voice. Some want more than this; maybe rocking them will help. If this does not calm your baby, try patting him on the back or rubbing his body. You may need to pick your baby up and quietly hold him against you. Some babies need to be gently rocked in your arms, either while you sit in a rocker or stand. At other times you may need to use all of these techniques: holding, rocking, singing, caressing, using eye contact, and speaking. Try each of these approaches, beginning with eye contact or speaking, until you find one that comforts your baby. (This is assuming, of course, that your baby is not crying from hunger, dampness, cold, or pain.)

The following question always comes up: "If I pay attention to my baby every time he cries, won't that spoil him?" Remember that it takes nine months of intrauterine growth before a baby is ready to be born. After the baby's birth, it takes at least nine more months of growth before he is somewhat independent. By then he is eating solid food, crawling, and grasping.

Babies require close physical contact before birth, and still need a great deal of contact after birth. A baby's crying can get on everyone's nerves, especially the parents. Everyone will be happier if you soothe your newborn when he cries. Do not worry about spoiling him. By taking care of his needs in infancy, you will teach him that the world is a friendly place with loving people. Your baby will not need to cry to develop his lungs. By letting him cry, all you will do is teach him that his needs will not be taken care of and that the world is hostile and uncaring. Studies have shown that children who were comforted when they cried as infants are significantly less demanding and fussy than children who were allowed to cry. Soothe your baby when he cries. This will stop most of his fussy crying during infancy, and will soothe your nerves later when he is older.

In addition to the previously discussed reasons for crying, some infants have a time every day during which they are fussy. This may occur at any time, day or night, and may drive the parents to distraction, because nothing seems to stop this crying. Sometimes this fussing only lasts for a couple of hours. This is called "periodic irritable crying." Other babies are fussy or cry hard for most of the day or night. This is sometimes caused by **colic**. Some feel that colic may be caused by an allergy to milk (caused by formula or by dairy products ingested by the nursing mother), or by an immature digestive system, because the baby appears to double up and cry with abdominal cramps. Comfort measures include those geared to relieve abdominal pain. Try laying the baby over your knees with his head and feet lower than his body, or laying the baby on his back and moving his legs in a bicycle-like fashion. Warmth or a circular massage of the abdomen may also help. You might also try carrying the baby on your hip, with his upper body hanging forward over your arm. This not only seems to soothe babies, but also allows them to see what is going on while freeing the mother's hands.

Other things you can do to comfort a fussy baby include swaddling the baby tightly in a blanket, rocking him in an automatic swing or cradle, placing him on a lamb's wool pad, or carrying him in a front baby carrier. A good comfort measure for the parents is a baby sitter, who can relieve the pressure on them for a few hours.

Another feeling parents often experience is anxiety. Because their child is so small and delicate, many parents are afraid that they may hurt him. Newborns are very flexible. Most of their skeletal structure has not yet developed into firm bone, but is composed of very tough, somewhat pliable cartilage. You needn't treat your baby like porcelain. He is "guaranteed not to break under normal conditions."

Another common feeling of new parents—especially mothers—is depression. This can be very upsetting, especially if you don't understand why you are crying. You may look at your new baby and at his proud father, and think that your happiness should be complete. Why, then, are you crying?

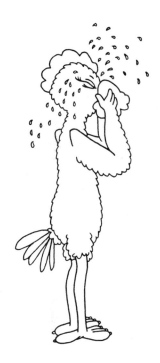

There are many possible causes for this depression, which is often called "baby blues." Profound hormonal changes occur after birth as your body returns to a nonpregnant state. This may play a major role in rapid mood fluctuations. In addition, while the changes that occur during pregnancy are gradual, the transition after birth is sudden. Overnight you will have a new body, and you may not like the way you look and feel. Your abdomen will be smaller, but it will still be flabby, and very few of your clothes will fit. Your breasts may be swollen and sore, and they may leak milk. If you had an episiotomy, you may have difficulty sitting and walking. You may not feel attractive and may dread the thought of intercourse. You may not look or feel like the person you used to be, and this can be depressing.

There will also be a drastic change in your role, especially if this will be your first child. You will no longer be carefree. Suddenly you will be a woman with awesome duties and responsibilities. Since the father will probably be gone most of the day, the main burden of caring for the baby will be yours. You will soon realize that caring for a new baby is a 24-hour-a-day job! New babies do sleep a lot, but they are awake and crying at the most inconvenient times. Your whole day will be filled with either caring for the baby or anticipating his care. You will have little time, if any, for yourself. The realization of this fact often comes as a severe shock to the new mother. You may wonder, "What have I done to myself?" and may begin to feel trapped and resentful of your child's intrusion into your life.

If this will not be your first child, you may be somewhat prepared for parenthood, but it will at some point become apparent that each new baby significantly increases the demands on your time. The other children will want your attention, and need to be reassured of your continuing love for them. They may become jealous of the time you spend with the new baby. They may even exhibit infantile behavior in order to get you to spend more time with them. An older child may begin to wet his pants again, want to sleep in a crib, or ask to drink from a bottle and be spoon-fed. This can be frustrating, but usually passes fairly quickly. (Refer to the chapter "Here We Go Again" on page 161.)

Fathers may also experience jealousy and resentment. They sometimes feel that the mother is spending so much time with the baby that she either has no time for them or is too tired to spend time with them. Mothers, also, may resent the time they spend with the baby and not with the father, or the fact that they have to "do it all," while he goes out and "has fun" (at work?).

Depression is closely related to fatigue. The deepest, most effective sleep usually occurs between six and seven hours after you go to sleep. Your new baby may cry every three to four hours for quite a while, so it will be very difficult for you to get a six- to seven-hour stretch of undisturbed sleep. A newborn's cry cannot be easily ignored, and nature intended that for his survival. But someone has to get up and care for the infant. This produces fatigue.

When you are tired, you are more easily irritated by situations that would not bother you at all if you were well rested. One possible solution is to have the baby sleep nearby. If you are going to nurse, you might plan to sleep with the baby. This will allow you to wake for the feedings and then drift back to sleep, relatively undisturbed by the interruption. Your baby can sleep with you all night or be returned to his crib sometime between feedings. You will not roll over and smother your baby. A normal newborn makes quite a fuss when his breathing is in any way hampered. You will surely wake up!

One common cause of fatigue is the visitor who drops in to see the new baby. He will seem to come most often when you are lying down to rest while the baby sleeps, and when the house is a mess because you have not had the time or energy to clean. You might try putting a sign on the door requesting that visitors call back later: "Baby is sleeping," or "Mom is resting. Please call later."

Eventually these things may make you angry—angry at visitors for coming when the house is a mess and you want to rest; angry at the new baby for his constant demands; angry at the other children for not behaving better and for requiring so much of your time; and angry at your husband for not helping you more, or not understanding your situation. You may then begin to feel guilty, because it really is not everyone else's fault that you are not reacting to the situation as you think you should. You may see other women handling the situation well, and feel that you can not even begin to get organized. You may begin to wonder "What is the matter with me? Am I going crazy?" You may become more angry, guilty, and finally miserably depressed.

Not every woman experiences jealousy, anger, and depression. Some are very fortunate and altogether avoid these unpleasant emotions, while others experience them only fleetingly. Perhaps they are receiving adequate rest because of help from friends or relatives, or perhaps they have their priorities arranged so that they will not become upset by the many little things that can go wrong. But women in ideal situations with wonderfully relaxed personalities and well-ordered priorities can still become depressed. It is important to keep in mind that this highly stressful situation is temporary and will disappear. Your body will adjust to its nonpregnant state, the baby will sleep longer at night, and you will get more rest. You will probably work out some routine with your husband and other children, and will adjust to the role of motherhood and really begin to enjoy your new life.

Although fathers rarely experience depression after birth, they also go through some difficult times after a baby is born. Besides having to make adjustments in lifestyle and role—with the responsibility of another person to feed, clothe, house, and educate—your life will be full of inconveniences. You will be able to get out of the house by going to work, but will not always be able to enjoy your time off. You will have to live with an unpredictable, sometimes irritable woman and a crying baby. Many parents do not enjoy a meal in peace for six months.

Every time you do something, you will first have to think of what to do with the baby. You will not be able to just "get up and go" anymore. When you finally make satisfactory arrangements for the baby, it will still take an additional half hour or more to get ready, so you may be late for everything. Sometimes it will become such a hassle to go out that you will find yourselves staying at home more. But that is no fun either, because your wife may be ignoring you and spending all her time with "that kid of hers," who seems to be crying all the time.

You may not understand your wife's feelings for the baby. After all, she is supposed to love you too. You may view your child as an intruder who is fouling up your whole life. Even your lovemaking attempts may be rejected because it hurts, or she is too tired, or the baby is crying. The spontaneity will be gone from your lives, and you may both feel trapped. These feelings do not occur in every family, but when they do exist, life at home is no fun.

There are two things that may be done to help relieve the tensions. First, get out of the situation; second, share the workload. Put up with the bother of going out; you may feel less trapped if you do. Get away from everything and spend some time together. Have a baby sitter care for the infant for a couple of hours. For this short time, his needs can be met by someone other than his parents.

Take time to focus on your relationship as a couple. Everyone in the family is affected when the parents are not on friendly terms. Being friends takes time. It cannot be achieved in the few quick minutes at the breakfast table when everyone is in a hurry or is hungry and irritable. Nor will the few minutes spent alone after the children are asleep—before you fade out from exhaustion—maintain the quality of your marriage. Make a date to do something special without the children at least twice a month. This does not have to be expensive; try going for a walk, and end the evening with an ice cream cone or sundae. Maybe each of you could make some suggestions, put them in a box, and pick one out every week. Consider this special time—*for the two of you alone.*

Some fathers are reluctant to assume some of the care of a newborn, perhaps because they do not understand the benefits they may derive from doing so. However, your feelings of abandonment may be decreased if you help with the baby, because your wife will then not be constantly alone with the child; you will be sharing that time. You will then also get to know your child sooner. Many fathers do not feel love for their child until the infant "becomes a person" and responds to them by smiling or talking. It is difficult to accept the inconveniences a new baby imposes upon a family when you feel indifferent or negative toward that baby. By caring

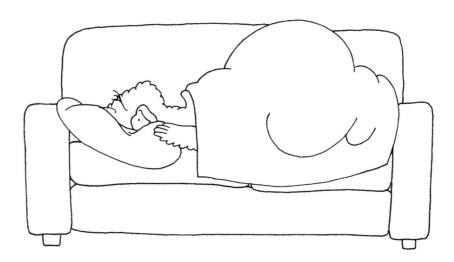

for the baby from early infancy, you will develop a more positive relationship with your child, and your life will be happier. In addition, your wife will have more time for you, as two people can often do things faster than one person. You will then be able to spend the time saved together.

You mothers should be particularly conscientious about fulfilling your own needs. You will not be able to meet the needs of the other family members until your needs are met. First, get as much rest as you can while the baby sleeps. You will be less irritable and depressed. Second, take care of yourself. Take time to wash your face, brush your teeth, comb your hair, and dress. Borrow or buy yourself at least two outfits that fit you.

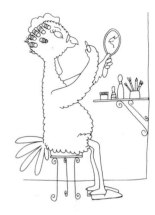

Third, do some exercises to get back in shape. During the first week after birth, do the Kegel exercises (see pages 33–34). To tone the abdomen, lie on the floor or bed with your legs bent, raise your head up, and hold it for a while; then lower your head. During the second week you can add the pelvic rock (see page 34). In the third week, add the "over and out" exercise (see page 35). Do each exercise ten times a day.

Make sure that you are eating a good diet composed of wholesome foods. The temptation is to just eat something, anything, in a hurry. Frequently this "something" is junk food, with lots of sugar but few nutrients. Try to eat plenty of fresh fruits and vegetables, whole grain breads and cereals, and meat and dairy products. Make time to do these things. You should feel mentally and physically refreshed as you do something to improve your appearance and health.

You cannot expect to be a perfect parent and a perfect housekeeper at the same time. Both you and your spouse may have to change your values, especially if this is your first child. Forget about your housework, and remember that with a new baby around, even cooking a simple meal can be a monumental task. Take advantage of frozen dinners and other easily prepared foods, take-out foods, and restaurants. Prepare in advance for hectic days. When you make a meal, double the quantity, and freeze the excess for a later date. Plan to use paper plates and plastic utensils.

If a diaper service is available in your area, consider using it for the first few months. Often this is cheaper than disposable diapers, and, of course, it is more convenient than doing your own. Either pay for the service yourself, or suggest that others give you gift certificates that apply toward the diaper service.

When friends or relatives offer their help, do not be too proud or independent to accept it. Let them make a meal or help with your laundry, housekeeping, shopping, or other tasks.

You may feel just wonderful right after your baby is born and be eager to resume your daily activities, but resist plunging into your old routine. For a while you will do fine, but suddenly you may find yourself overwhelmed and exhausted. It may help to remind yourself that having a baby is physically and emotionally draining. Your body's need for rest can be masked by this short burst of energy and exhilaration. Consider the first couple weeks of your new baby's life as a vacation for the whole family, during which you will not do much beyond the bare necessities. This will be a time for getting adjusted to your new situation.

Many families arrange to have someone come in to help out after the baby is born. There are many pros and cons to this. Sometimes the person who comes in to help becomes a guest requiring your attention. You may find yourself worrying about the helper's needs, or socializing with her instead of resting. Other helpers may take over the care of the baby, leaving you with the housekeeping tasks. Either of these situations will affect the family's adjustment—usually by delaying it. Consider having the father take some time off from work. This can be a very intimate time of sharing, and both of you will feel more comfortable learning to care for your newborn together. If someone else is coming to help, let her help by cleaning house, baby sitting for the older children, and preparing meals, while you spend time resting and getting acquainted with your baby and each other.

After you have adjusted to the new baby and your new life, new concerns will appear. Are you raising your child properly? Where are his teeth? Why isn't he walking? Perhaps you should feed him more vegetables, meat, or fruit (or you are feeding him too much vegetables, meat, or fruit). When are you going to toilet train your child? Why does he cry so much? You should do this or that—you should *not* do this or that. It is easy to be perfect parents before your baby is born, but not as easy afterwards. We suggest that you read as many books on child care as you can. If you read 12 books, you will get 12 different approaches. Then you can feel free to do whatever seems right to you, knowing that somewhere there exists an authority who supports your approach.

Another important thing to remember is that children go through pleasant and unpleasant stages of behavior. When your child is in a pleasant phase, you will have no doubts that you are raising him properly. He will seem perfect, and you will feel like wonderful parents. However, during temper tantrums and bouts of disobedience—times when your child is learning how to assert himself and be independent—you may feel like failures.

The goal of parenting is not the complete enjoyment of the child, but the creation of a responsible, happy adult. You probably will not know whether you have done a good job as parents until your child is fully grown, so do not worry now about what others say concerning your abilities as parents. Do whatever you feel is right for your child. Then you will be able to relax and enjoy your children. They will provide joy that is not possible in any other way. So, enjoy, enjoy, enjoy your children!

Career Choices

During World War II, women had to move into the work force. Many stayed there, while others began working in later years due to economic necessity.

Today, most women work outside the home before they have children, and expect to continue doing so afterwards. Somewhere along the line, women began believing that you have to work and be paid for that work. Nobody pays the mother at home. Since she does not get paid, she must not be working. While it may still be acceptable to stay at home while your children are very small, there is now great pressure to return to work as soon as possible, especially if you have any marketable skills. The option of staying home to raise your children is frequently not even considered.

You and your spouse should discuss your priorities. Try to decide what the physical and emotional needs of each member of your family are, and how they can best be met. These needs may change, and should be evaluated periodically. Your decision regarding work outside the home should be made after considering these needs.

One of the advantages of staying home to raise your children is that no one can raise a child with as much love and concern as you can. You can provide guidance and instill your own values into your children. You will be there to enjoy and appreciate every aspect of your child's growth. You will be an integral part of his life. Another advantage is that this will be a time spent away from your career—a time to work on your own personal growth. Skills you develop while raising your children will be valuable to you later if you return to the outside work force.

On the other hand, there are several advantages to working outside the home. The most obvious advantage is more money, and all the things that that money can provide. Another advantage is that you will receive some recognition for your efforts and a possible increase in your self-esteem. You will have an identity through your job—aside from being somebody's

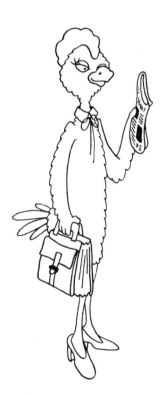

mother. If one day you do not go to work, you will be missed; and when you go and do a good job, you will be appreciated. Last, but not least, some of the less rewarding aspects of parenting, such as toilet training, can be delegated to others.

To make an informed choice, you must also consider the disadvantages of each of these situations. Loss of income is one of the disadvantages of staying home. You may feel guilty about depriving your family of extra material things. You may also find that the lack of recognition you receive for your efforts affects you. This will be especially obvious when, after a particularly difficult day with a sick two-year-old, someone asks, "Don't you work?" Parenting is not considered "work" by many people, because you do not get paid for it. This attitude can chip away at your self-esteem.

If you had a promising career before you had children, you may be concerned about re-entering the job market after the children are somewhat grown. You may also feel guilty about wasting your talents and skills. Being isolated in a house with little children may produce a craving for some adult conversation. You may find yourself waiting for the mailman so that you can say "hello" to him, or trying to get a conversation started with the grocery clerk.

On the other hand, there are also disadvantages to working outside the home. Traditionally, child care and homemaking tasks have been the woman's responsibility. In many homes in which both parents work outside the house, the mother finds that she still has most of the responsibility for the children and the home. A working woman often finds that she has little or no time for herself or for socializing with friends. She may feel guilty, as her many responsibilities prevent her from adequately attending to any of her tasks. She may worry especially about her relationship with her children, and may also feel concern about the quality of the care her children are receiving. The conflict is especially acute when children are sick, when children have special school programs, or when medical visits are scheduled during working hours. Sometimes the financial benefits are not as great as expected after deducting the costs of child care, transportation, clothing, meals, and other hidden expenses.

Are there any alternatives to these two choices? Yes! There are part-time jobs that leave you more time for your family, or jobs that can be done during the evenings on which your spouse is home. Increasing in popularity is the shared job, in which two people assume the responsibility for one job. They mutually decide how the hours and benefits should be divided.

Other women work in their homes, doing things they enjoy doing. You would be amazed at how many people will pay for your skills. Some examples of home-based jobs are child care, bookkeeping, typing, tutoring or teaching, telephone answering services, sewing, drawing, writing, catering, and computer programming. You may think of others. Decide what skills you have, and advertise.

Another alternative that is increasing in popularity is the arrangement in which the father becomes the at-home parent, while the mother works outside the home.

Parenting is not like any other job. There is no supervisor and no one to tell you if you are doing it wrong—but then no one tells you if you are doing it right, either. Once you get the hang of it, the technical skills are simple. The more difficult skills are emotional—meeting the needs of someone who is unable to give you a clear indication of what he needs, and supervising behavior. It is important to remember that parenting is a job, even though it is unpaid. The person taking care of the growth and development of children is utilizing many skills and talents for which she would be highly paid outside the home. However, she is also doing some very menial tasks for which the pay would not be as great.

There are many things to consider when deciding whether to work at home or outside the home, and what part each parent should play in the parenting process. A few hours spent identifying your needs, evaluating the available choices, or brainstorming for new solutions, will produce the best plan for your family. Hop to it!

Postpartum Sexual Adjustment

The birth of your baby will mark a new era in your life—a time of many changes during which you will adjust to the joys and demands of parenting. For many couples, the birth of a child brings about drastic changes in their sexual relationship—changes that may require some difficult adjustments. Some couples, having no problems in this area, may wonder at the need for the information included in this section. In fact, they may find it offensive. This section is not written for them. It is intended for those couples who are silently struggling with a problem that they may feel is unique to them. Perhaps they feel that there is no place to turn to for help, or perhaps they are too embarrassed by their failure to adjust to seek help, even if they do know where to find it. So they continue to struggle, wondering what is wrong with them. An explanation of the physical and emotional factors that sometimes contribute to sexual difficulties after birth can help them to realize they are not that unusual, and that these problems are common occurrences. It is quite normal to experience these things.

Even when the mother does not have an episiotomy, she may experience soreness in the perineal area. After an episiotomy, most birth attendants suggest refraining from intercourse until the episiotomy has healed. The pelvic floor (Kegel) exercises help to speed healing and increase comfort.

Even after the episiotomy has healed, many women find that pressure on the perineum is uncomfortable, or even painful. Intercourse, also, may be painful. This is not uncommon, and will diminish in time. Changing positions and using additional lubrication may increase comfort. Side-lying or woman-superior positions often put less pressure on the site of the episiotomy than does the man-superior position. These positions also give the woman more control over the direction and depth of penetration, which may help to eliminate the fear of her partner inadvertently hurting her. The man, too, may be relieved of the fear of hurting the woman when she has more control over the pressure placed on the perineum. Until ovulation occurs, vaginal lubrication may be decreased. The use of a water-based lubricant may be helpful.

Fatigue, also, may be a strong deterrent to lovemaking. Caring for a baby is hard work—often more difficult and time consuming than either parent imagined. By the time the mother finally gets the baby to bed, it is often sleep, and not sex, that is on her mind. It is difficult to make love when the woman is sleeping, and she may become downright irritable if awakened. Fathers can help by assisting with the chores and baby care. The mother should rest every day. Mothers must learn to ignore the demands of housekeeping, and to nap when the baby naps. If the baby has been fussy all day and the mother has not been able to take a nap, it may be a good idea for the father to hold down the fort for a while to give the mother time to rest. This may seem silly at six o'clock in the evening, but remember that a new mother's day often doesn't end until eleven or twelve o'clock. Letting the mother rest early in the evening may give her energy for lovemaking later on.

Once you do get over the hurdle and become involved in lovemaking, you may find it either disconcerting or funny to find yourselves taking a bath in breast milk. This is due to the oxytocin that is released during physical arousal, causing the milk to let down (see page 153). Nurse the baby to help him sleep and to lessen the likelihood of spraying milk.

The emotional overtones that may contribute to sexual problems are often more varied and difficult to deal with. These may include a preoccupation with the baby, frustration resulting from a lack of available time to spend together as a couple, and the fear of pregnancy.

Preoccupation with the baby takes various forms. All day, the mother races around the house, caring for the baby. When the father comes home, he too begins to concern himself with the baby's care. It is difficult to unwind and enjoy a rip-roaring sexual encounter at the end of the day. You may fear that the baby will awaken, cry, or disturb you in some way. (It is true that sometimes their timing is not very good!) A crying baby can be very inhibiting. Try to arrange your lovemaking at a time when the baby is less likely to disturb you. Feeding the baby, getting him to sleep, and then moving to another part of the house may help you to relax.

Many women are confused by their decreased sexual desire, and fear that their feelings are not normal. They find that they are perfectly happy with cuddling and kissing, and do not want to go any further. This may be due in part to the close relationship they have with their babies, which, to a great extent, fulfills their need for love and physical contact. It may also be due to the great demands the baby places on the mother. The mother may feel that she has so many demands on her during the day that when she goes to bed she just wants to be left alone. Sex may become another demand—another chore to be done.

This is a very difficult time for many couples. Two things may help. First, the partners should discuss their feelings openly and lovingly. The man may have to accept that cuddling does not always end in intercourse. This may be a good time to develop other ways of expressing love.

You will probably find that the time you have for romance is shorter than it was before the birth of your child. One possible solution is to schedule a time to be shared as husband and wife, instead of mom and dad. During the day, the mother should plan to get herself ready. Take time to bathe and do your hair. Spend the day thinking about your evening together. Organize your time so that you will not be tired at night. Let the house go, and either make dinner in the morning or arrange to have take-out food. Rest in the afternoon and be ready when your husband gets home.

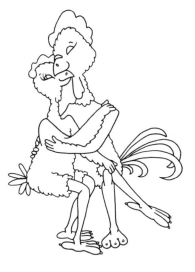

Fathers should plan to provide a loving atmosphere. Bring your wife a gift, and tell her how much she means to you and how much you care about her. While the baby is awake, play with him together. When he goes to sleep, have a quiet dinner and spend time holding, caressing, and kissing her. Do not rush. Give her time to unwind and become aware of how much you mean to her and how much she loves you. Once the romantic mood is set, sex may follow; however, your goal should not be sex, but time together. She may otherwise feel pressured and be unable to enjoy the evening. If at this time she does not want intercourse, perhaps she soon will. Your loving and caring attitude will do more to stir her sexual desire than anything else you can do.

Another problem regarding intercourse is the fear of pregnancy. The baby you have is wonderful, but you may not want another one right away. The proper use of a reliable birth control method will help to relieve that worry. The following chart from the United States Department of Health, Education, and Welfare may help in your choice of methods. Your birth attendant can also give you information.

METHODS OF CONTRACEPTION

Method	What Is It?	How Does It Work?	How Reliable or Effective Is It?
"The Pill"	Pills with two hormones, an estrogen and progestin, similar to the hormones a woman makes during pregnancy.	It prevents egg's release from woman's ovaries, makes cervical mucus thicker, and changes lining of the uterus.	99.7% if used consistently, but much less effective if used carelessly.
"Mini-Pills"	Pills with just one type of hormone: a progestin similar to a hormone a woman makes in her own ovaries.	It may prevent egg's release from woman's ovaries. Makes cervical mucus thicker and changes lining of uterus, making it harder for a fertilized egg to start growing there.	97%–99% if used correctly, but less effective if used carelessly.
Intrauterine Device (IUD)	A small piece of plastic with nylon threads attached. Some have copper wrapped around them. One IUD gives off the hormone progesterone.	The IUD is inserted into the uterus. It is not known exactly how the IUD prevents pregnancy.	95%–99% if patient checks for string regularly.

Eventually, the physical and emotional factors that are adversely affecting your postpartum love life will disappear. In the meantime, probably the greatest thing that will help you during this adjustment is a sense of humor. Being able to look at the funny side of a situation will be of great assistance—not only in the bedroom, but in every room of your house—while you are experiencing the "joys" of parenthood.

How Would I Use It?	Are There Problems With It?	What Are the Side Effects or Complications?	What Are the Advantages?
Either of two ways: 1. A pill a day for 3 weeks, stop for 1 week, then start a new pack. 2. A pill every single day with no stopping between packs.	Must be prescribed by a doctor. All women should have medical exam before taking the pill, and some women should not take it.	Nausea, weight gain, headaches, missed periods, darkened skin on the face, breast tenderness, or depression may occur. More serious and more rare problems are blood clots in the legs, the lungs, or the brain, and heart attacks. Do not use if nursing.	Convenient, extremely effective, does not interfere with sex, and may diminish menstrual cramps.
Take one pill every single day as long as you want to avoid pregnancy.	Must be prescribed by a doctor. All women should have a medical exam first.	Irregular periods, missed periods, and spotting may occur, and are more common problems with mini-pills than with the regular birth control pills.	Convenient, effective, does not interfere with sex, and has less serious side effects than do regular birth control pills.
Check string at least once a month right after your period ends to make sure your IUD is still properly in place.	Must be inserted by a doctor after a pelvic examination. Cannot be used by all women. Sometimes the uterus "pushes" it out.	May cause cramps, bleeding, or spotting. Infections of the uterus or the Fallopian tubes may be serious. See a doctor for pain, bleeding, fever, or a foul-smelling discharge. Nursing mothers may experience cramping, heavier discharge, and/or expulsion of the IUD.	Effective, always there when needed, and usually not felt by either partner.

METHODS OF CONTRACEPTION—*Continued*

Method	What Is It?	How Does It Work?	How Reliable or Effective Is It?
Diaphragm with Spermicidal Jelly or Cream	A shallow rubber cup used with a sperm-killing jelly or cream.	The diaphragm fits inside the vagina. The rubber cup forms a barrier between the uterus and the sperm. The jelly or cream kills the sperm.	About 97% effective if used correctly and consistently, but much less effective if used carelessly.
Spermicidal Foam, Jelly, or Cream	Cream and jelly come in tubes; foam comes in aerosol cans or individual applicators. Is placed in vagina.	Foam, jelly and cream contain a chemical that kills sperm and acts as a physical barrier between sperm and uterus.	About 90%–97% effective if used correctly and consistently, but much less effective if used carelessly.
Condom ("Rubber")	A sheath of rubber shaped to fit snugly over the erect penis.	It prevents sperm from getting inside a woman's vagina during intercourse.	About 97% effective if used correctly and consistently, but much less effective if used carelessly.
Condom and Foam Used Together		It prevents sperm from getting inside the uterus by killing sperm and by preventing sperm from getting out into the vagina.	Close to 100% effective if both foam and condoms are used with every act of intercourse.

How Would I Use It	Are There Problems With It?	What Are the Side Effects or Complications?	What Are the Advantages?
Insert the diaphragm and jelly (or cream) before intercourse. Must be inserted no earlier than 2 hours before intercourse. Must stay in place at least 8 hours after intercourse.	Must be fitted by a doctor after a pelvic exam. Some women find it difficult to insert, inconvenient, or messy. Refittings required after pregnancy or weight loss.	Some women find that the jelly or cream irritates the vagina. Try changing brands if this occurs.	Effective and safe.
Put foam, jelly, or cream into your vagina each time you have intercourse, not more than 30 minutes beforehand. No douching for at least 8 hours after intercourse.	Must be inserted just before intercourse. Some find it inconvenient or messy.	Some women find that the foam, cream, or jelly irritates the vagina. May irritate the man's penis. Try changing brands if this happens.	Effective, safe, a good lubricant, and can be purchased in a drugstore.
The condom should be placed on the erect penis before the penis comes into contact with the vagina. After ejaculation, the penis should be removed from the vagina immediately.	Objectionable to some men and women. Interrupts intercourse. May be messy. Condom may break.	A few individuals are allergic to rubber. If this is a problem, condoms called "skins," which are not made of rubber, are available.	Effective, safe, can be purchased in a drugstore. Excellent protection against sexually transmitted infections.
Foam must be inserted within 30 minutes before intercourse, and condom must be placed on erect penis prior to contact with vagina.	Requires more effort than some couples like. May be messy or inconvenient. Interrupts intercourse.	No serious complications.	Extremely effective, safe, and both items may be purchased in a drugstore without a doctor's prescription. Excellent protection against sexually transmitted infections.

METHODS OF CONTRACEPTION—*Continued*

Method	What Is It?	How Does It Work?	How Reliable or Effective Is It?
Periodic Abstinence (Natural Family Planning)	Ways of finding out days each month when you are most likely to get pregnant. Intercourse is avoided at that time.	Techniques include maintaining chart of basal body temperature, checking vaginal secretions, and keeping calendar of menstrual periods, all of which can help predict when you are most likely to release an egg.	Certain methods are about 90%–97% effective if used consistently. Other methods are less effective. Combining techniques increases effectiveness.
Sterilization	Vasectomy (male); tubal ligation (female). Ducts carrying sperm or egg are tied and cut surgically.	The closing of tubes in male prevents sperm from reaching egg; the closing of tubes in female prevents egg from reaching sperm.	Almost 100% effective and *not* usually reversible.

How Would I Use It	Are There Problems With It?	What Are the Side Effects or Complications?	What Are the Advantages?
Careful records must be maintained of several factors: basal body temperature, vaginal secretions, and onset of menstrual periods. Careful study of these methods will dictate when intercourse should be avoided.	Difficult to use if menstrual cycle is irregular. Sexual intercourse must be avoided for a significant part of each cycle.	No complications.	Safe and effective if followed carefully. Little if any religious objection to method. Teaches women about their menstrual cycle.
After the decision to have no more children has been well thought through, a brief surgical procedure is performed on the man or the woman.	Surgical operation has some risk, but serious complications are rare. Sterilization should not be performed unless no more children are desired.	All surgical operations have some risk, but serious complications are uncommon. Some pain may last for several days. Rarely, the wrong structure is tied off, or the tube grows back together. There is no loss of sexual desire or ability in vast majority of patients.	The most effective method. Low rate of complications. Many feel that removing fear of pregnancy improves sexual relations.

Chapter Six
Feeding Your Baby

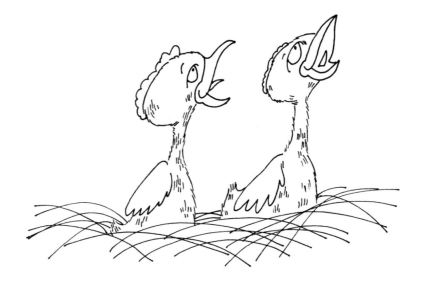

There are many important decisions to make during your pregnancy. What color should I paint the nursery? Which infant seat should I buy? What type of crib should I get? Should I use cloth or paper diapers? Should grandma come to help? These are all important. But the decision about how to feed your baby, although it is even more important, is often based on little or no information.

There are two methods of infant feeding, breast and bottle. Sometimes a mother chooses to bottle feed her baby simply because her friend did and, "Honestly, I haven't thought much about it, but I suppose I will too." Since a number of women still choose to bottle feed without seriously considering breastfeeding, we would like to list the advantages and disadvantages of nursing so that you can understand more about it, and make an informed decision regarding the feeding method that is best for you. The American Academy of Pediatrics has recommended that its members encourage breastfeeding among their patients because breast milk is best for the baby during his first year. The following information will tell you why.

THE ADVANTAGES OF BREASTFEEDING

Benefits for the Baby

Human milk is the perfect food for human babies. Milks vary in composition from species to species, and seem to reflect the needs of each species. For example, calves double their birth weight in one-third the time that human babies do, and we find that cow's milk contains three times more protein than human milk.

One obvious difference between human newborns and the offspring of other mammals is their length of dependency. Calves begin feeding and moving with the herd within a few days after birth. It takes about nine to twelve months before the human baby can move about unaided and feed himself. This reflects differences in brain development at birth. Human milk is especially suited for human brain growth.

The composition of breast milk changes as the baby gets older and his needs change. There is more protein and fat in the milk produced after birth than in that produced six months after birth. There are also variations in the milk composition during each day. The milk at night has more fat than the milk in the morning, perhaps enabling the baby to sleep longer at night.

The vitamin and mineral content of breast milk is different from that of cow's milk, which forms the base of most infant formulas. Although there is little iron in breast milk, anemia is rare in breast-fed babies. Perhaps all the iron in breast milk is utilized more efficiently because all elements necessary for the absorption of iron are available in breast milk. There is more cholesterol in human milk, and some evidence suggests that early exposure to cholesterol increases the body's ability to control cholesterol levels later in life. Every investigation into the composition of breast milk shows more constituents that are important for the baby's health and well-being, with none of them altered or destroyed during processing (as with formula).

During the first couple of days after birth, an early milk substance, called **colostrum**, is produced by the mother. Colostrum is mostly protein, and contains antibodies to protect the baby from diseases. Colostrum also appears to coat the baby's intestines, thus preventing harmful bacteria and allergy-producing proteins from entering the baby's system. Human breast milk has been used to treat epidemics of newborn infectious diarrhea. Almost every mechanism in the body used to treat infection is present in breast milk. Studies show that formula-fed infants have two to three times more respiratory and gastrointestinal infections and hospitalizations for these infections than breast-fed babies, especially when the breast-fed babies have been nursed for four to five months. During pregnancy, the baby receives antibodies to many infectious diseases through the placenta. These immunities last for several months after birth. The breast-fed infant continues to receive these passive immunities for as long as he is nursed.

Breast-fed babies have better teeth, better palate development, and fewer cavities than bottle-fed babies. This is due to the different position of their mouths and the alignment of their jaws as they suck to obtain milk. They also do not fall asleep with milk in their mouths, because they continue to suck and swallow after the breast has been emptied of milk. Studies have shown that formula-fed babies are heavier than breast-fed babies. We used to think that this was healthy, but excessive weight gain in infancy has now been associated with obesity in later life. This increased weight may be due to the fact that formula is often made richer than recommended, and that the adult, not the infant, controls his food intake. There is a tendency to encourage the baby to finish the bottle, even when the infant has had enough. Solid foods are often started sooner, too, when the baby has been formula-fed.

Constipation is rare in breast-fed infants because the milk is rapidly and easily digested. The infant's stool is soft, and may vary in frequency from several times a day to once every several days. Do not be concerned if your baby does not have a stool every day as long as, when he does, it is soft. The stools of breast-fed babies are not as offensive in odor and do not stain as badly as formula stools. They are frequently a golden yellow color, but may change color according to the mother's diet, especially if she eats broccoli or other highly colored foods.

Physical Benefits for the Mother

About six to seven pounds of the weight gain of pregnancy is composed of extra fat deposits that provide the mother with extra calories during early lactation. This weight may remain if the mother does not nurse or diet after her baby's birth. Nursing also helps the uterus return to its pre-pregnant state sooner. When the baby nurses, the hormone oxytocin is released to produce a milk let-down (see page 153). Oxytocin functions as a tranquilizer in the mother's body. A woman who feels insecure about raising her child may benefit from this phenomenon, as well as from the knowledge that she can meet her infant's needs.

Nursing a baby also forces the mother to rest. She cannot nurse while vacuuming, washing, cooking, or scrubbing. She cannot prop her breast on a pillow and leave. She must sit or lie down. This is a definite advantage for the new mother, who may feel so good that she overexerts herself.

Emotional Benefits for the Mother

Many mothers who breastfeed their babies say that they feel extraordinarily close to their infants. Nursing produces a symbiotic relationship. The baby needs milk and the mother needs to give milk. Often mothers awaken at night just before the infant does. Mother and child seem to be closely in tune. Words fail to describe the feelings of love, joy, pride, completeness, and competence a mother feels as she holds her infant to her breast.

Convenience

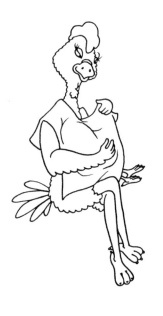

There are many who feel that nursing a baby is too much work. Not so! Think of how convenient it would be to have your baby's food always available, warm, and sterile—especially when he wakes from hunger at 3:00 A.M. You won't have to wait for the formula to warm up while he screams and awakens the whole family. All you need do is nurse him in bed with you. You will not even have to fully wake up. Do not be afraid of smothering the baby. A healthy baby will wiggle and nudge you or your blankets off his face.

If you nurse your child, there will be no need to sterilize milk containers or nipples. You will be able to take your baby anywhere and stay as long as you like without worrying about how much formula should be taken along and how it can be kept from spoiling while you are gone. All you will need is a supply of clean diapers.

You will always be able to nurse your baby discreetly if you have a blanket to put over your shoulder and wear clothes that pull up from the waist or unbutton from the bottom. If your baby is full but still fussy, the breast will act as a pacifier; a bottle would not help at all.

Economy

Formula will add $5.00 to $20.00 to your weekly budget, but extra nutrition for the mother may only add $4.00 to $6.00 per week. Because breast milk contains about 40 calories per ounce, and the mother's body has to work to make milk, the mother should eat about 1,000 extra calories a day. This can be fun—surely better than dieting.

THE DISADVANTAGES OF BREASTFEEDING

Only the Mother Can Breastfeed the Baby

The fact that the mother alone is responsible for the baby's nourishment may be a disadvantage in your family situation, especially if you have to return to work soon after your baby is born. If you do plan to work and nurse, make sure to breastfeed just before leaving; at lunch time, if possible; and after you return from work. Perhaps you can have your sitter refrain from feeding him for one hour before your expected return. Of course, if you are going to be late you had better call, or all will be chaos when you arrive.

To avoid problems, decide in advance how the baby is to be fed when you are not there to nurse him. He can have breast milk that you expressed at an earlier time (see pages 153–154), formula, or—if he is of the appropriate age—solid foods. The decision is yours. One factor to keep in mind is that the less your baby nurses, the less milk you will produce. Consequently, if you intend to nurse him for a long period of time, you will have to nurse him frequently.

Frequent Feedings

The breast-fed baby may nurse every two to four hours. Cow's milk, which is the base of most infant formulas, produces a larger curd which remains in the stomach longer, making the baby feel full longer. Breast milk is digested more quickly, and the baby becomes hungry sooner. Do not worry about a feeding schedule. Sometimes your baby will want to nurse after one hour; then, perhaps, not for another five hours. Your nursing baby may begin sleeping through the night just as soon as a formula-fed baby would.

Longer Feedings

Your breast-fed baby will get about 90 percent of the milk during the first seven minutes. However, he may continue to suck for up to a half an hour longer, and you will not know if he is still drinking or not. When bottle feeding, you can see when the bottle is empty, and the baby stops sucking when he begins to take in air. Also, milk comes out of the bottle more easily and with less effort than it does from the breast, thus shortening the feeding time.

Sore Nipples

Often, the mother's nipples become sore after the baby has been nursing for a short time. This problem sometimes causes the mother to wean her child earlier than intended. The problem of sore nipples can be avoided or lessened by preparing the nipples for nursing during the last two months of pregnancy (see page 152) and slowly increasing the baby's time at each breast from five to fifteen minutes. Nipple soreness does not normally occur after the first four weeks of the breastfeeding relationship.

Sibling Rivalry

Some mothers are reluctant to nurse a second baby, fearing that the older children will be jealous. Actually, you can spend your nursing time very productively by reading stories and talking and listening to your older children. You will be their captive audience. You will not get up and do chores, and will still have one arm free to cuddle your older child.

Exclusion of the Father

The father, or other family members, may want to feed the baby. Remember that there are many other ways in which the family can interact with the baby. Family members can enjoy playing with, cuddling, changing, bathing, talking to, and caressing the baby. The more physical contact your baby gets, the more content he is likely to be.

Discomfort During Intercourse

Nursing usually prevents ovulation, which is the release of the egg from the ovary that occurs at about the middle of the menstrual cycle. Until ovulation takes place, the vaginal secretions are decreased. You may be aroused sexually but have no vaginal lubrication. This dryness will make intercourse uncomfortable, but can be easily overcome with the use of a water-based lubricant such as K-Y Jelly. Be aware that although ovulation usually does not occur when you nurse, it can. Do not use breastfeeding as a means of contraception.

MAKING A DECISION

Both your feelings and those of your partner are very important when making a decision about whether to breastfeed or bottle feed your child. Breastfeeding is not something just the mother does; it involves the support and encouragement of the whole family. Breastfeeding is an intensely personal event, and you should not feel guilty about a decision not to nurse. Sometimes nursing is impossible. Forcing yourself to breastfeed when you feel uncomfortable about it will not be good for you or your baby. Breastfeeding is just one act of mothering. If you feel resentful each time you think of or attempt to nurse, are tense because the nursing relationship deprives you of time that could be spent with other family members, or must work, etc., it may be best for you to bottle feed your baby. Today's formulas closely duplicate human milk, and have successfully nourished thousands, if not millions, of babies. More than a method of feeding, nursing is a means of communication. Some women may communicate more positive feelings of love and acceptance if they bottle feed their infants. By holding, caressing, and talking to your baby while he drinks his bottle and allowing him to stop when he is full, you will provide your baby with both nourishment and love.

BREASTFEEDING

Get Ready . . .

Beginning in the seventh or eighth month of pregnancy, you should start preparing your nipples for nursing. One way is to hand express a few drops of colostrum daily. To do so, place your thumb at the top edge of the areola (the dark ring around the nipple), and your middle finger at the bottom of the areola. Squeeze gently, sliding your fingers toward the nipple. Then rotate your hand slightly, squeeze and slide again, and repeat. You might try doing this in a warm shower.

Leave your breasts exposed to air or to the friction of clothing for a while each day. You can do this by lowering the flaps of a nursing bra, or by going braless. You can also rub your nipples gently with a washcloth during a bath or shower, or gently tug, roll, or stimulate them during lovemaking. Nursing is a pleasant experience, so do not get compulsive about breast preparation. It, too, should be pleasant.

Get Set . . .

There are a few things to keep in mind when you begin nursing your newborn. First, you should nurse your baby as soon as possible after birth. Sometimes the first feeding is disappointing, because the baby may not take hold and suck vigorously. Many babies are just not hungry after birth, and are content to simply lick and explore the nipple. When he is hungry, he will nurse.

Nurse your baby "on demand"—either when he is hungry or when you need to nurse your baby. Some babies need to suck often. Yours may suck his fingers, or you may choose to give him a pacifier or allow him to nurse frequently. Nurse on both breasts at each feeding, beginning with the breast you ended with at the last feeding. As a reminder, place a pin on your bra, indicating the side on which you last nursed. After a while you will feel which breast is fuller, and will begin with that breast.

Initially, you may want to nurse just a couple of minutes on each breast, gradually increasing the time to satisfy the needs of your baby. Babies are born with a **rooting reflex**—an instinct necessary for their survival. The rooting reflex is stimulated when the baby's cheek is stroked, either with a finger or the nipple. Your baby will turn to the direction of the stroked cheek with his mouth open wide (like a hungry baby bird). The time will then be right to place as much of the areola into the baby's mouth as possible. To break the suction when ending a nursing session, do not pull the baby off the nipple. Place a finger into the corner of the baby's mouth and gently release the pressure created by the baby's sucking. Sore nipples may result from pulling the baby off the nipple.

Go . . .

While you are nursing, make sure that you eat a good, balanced diet and plenty of fluids. You will not have to drink milk to make milk; juice or water will do. When you sit down to nurse your baby, take a glass of something to drink with you. Make sure that you and your baby are comfortable. If necessary, use pillows for support. At night you can nurse in bed. Just lie on your side and expose your breast; the baby will find it, nurse, and then go back to sleep.

When you begin nursing, the baby will suck a little before you feel a tingling sensation in your breasts. This is the **let-down reflex**. It occurs when the milk is being squeezed out of the ducts. When the milk begins to let down, press your hand against the nipple that the baby is not using. This will prevent milk from leaking out of that nipple.

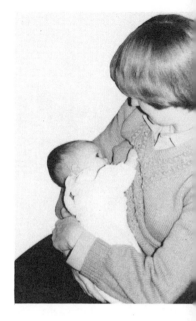

Hold your baby "belly to belly" while nursing.

Expressing and Storing Milk

If you want to express milk to freeze it for later use, hold a sterile cup under the breast that's not being nursed at, instead of pressing the breast. You can speed this process by expressing the milk as you did during pregnancy (see page 152). You will usually be able to express more milk during the first morning feeding than you will during later feedings. Place the expressed milk in a sterile bottle, seal, and freeze. The frozen milk should keep for about two weeks. Do not defrost it until you are ready to use it.

Breast milk is watery in appearance. When frozen, the cream separates from the milk because the milk is not homogenized. Freeze the milk in a small, four-ounce bottle rather than a large, eight-ounce bottle, because there will then be less chance of wasting this precious fluid. When you leave the house, take out as many bottles of milk as you think the baby sitter will need. In the first month you may have more milk than your baby needs, so freeze the excess. Later, the supply will adjust to your baby's demands.

Breast Care

Keep your breasts clean and dry. Simply washing them with warm water is sufficient under normal circumstances. Unless you have sore breasts, you should not use lotions or creams.

Sore nipples are common during the first month or so. They are not only uncomfortable, but may predispose you to infections and make your baby cranky. To help prevent and relieve this soreness, keep your nipple exposed to the air daily for short periods of time. You can purchase a two-piece plastic shield—one that has an air space—to wear inside your bra to keep your clothing off the nipples and to help the nipples stay dry. Pure hydrous lanolin or Vitamin E oil applied after each nursing may also help. You will not have to wash these substances off. Do not use soap or alcohol on the breast or plastic liners in your bra, as these tend to cause sore nipples by keeping the breasts either too dry or too moist.

If your nipples are sore, check the position of the baby's mouth when he nurses. He should have not just the nipple, but also a good amount of the dark area around the nipple (the areola) in his mouth. Sore nipples can also be caused by improper body positioning. When nursing, your baby should be facing you "belly-to-belly." He should not have to turn his head to nurse. You can position him properly by sitting up, lying on your side with the baby lying next to you, lying on your back with the baby on you, or supporting the baby in a football hold with his face forward and his body under your arm.

If you are tense, your let-down reflex may be delayed, and your baby may begin gnawing on the nipple in frustration. Try taking a warm shower before the baby's feeding time or drinking something soothing (warm milk or herbal tea) as the baby nurses.

Plugged ducts occur when the breast has not been sufficiently emptied, and milk plugs one of the ducts in the nipple. You may notice a small white dot on the nipple (do not try to rub this off, as it is beneath the skin), or you may find that a section of the breast feels hard because the milk has not been drained from that section. The breast may feel full, hot, and sore, and the nipple may hurt as the baby nurses.

The best way of treating a sore breast is to empty the breast completely. You may find it helpful to stay in bed with your baby and apply moist heat to the affected area. Keep a supply of diapers, plenty of fluids, and a good book nearby. Relax, and consider this a vacation day. Pamper yourself, and nurse your baby often. If only one breast is sore, have the baby nurse on the unaffected side until you feel the milk let down; then switch to the sore side. His sucking will then be more gentle, because the milk will be flowing smoothly. If both breasts are sore, it may help to massage the breast from the chest wall toward the nipple and express some milk before nursing. This is especially effective when done in the shower.

Breast infections can produce the same symptoms as plugged ducts, with either the whole breast or part of the breast feeling hard from **engorgement** (overfilled breasts). Sometimes the breasts are not hard, red, or painful, but, instead, you have a fever and feel miserable. If you have flu-like symptoms or red, hot, and sore breasts, contact your doctor. He may prescribe antibiotics. In most cases the best treatment is to keep the breasts as empty as possible. Again, bed rest, moist heat, plenty of fluids, and frequent nursing help.

Often the question comes up about whether the baby is getting enough nourishment. If your baby wets his diaper six times a day, he is getting enough. Babies grow at different rates, and the rate of growth is largely affected by heredity. There is a wide range of normal heights and weights. Nursing babies eat more often than formula-fed babies, as indicated earlier. This is perfectly normal. They also have growth spurts at about one month and three months, although this may vary. During growth spurts, your baby will want to eat more often. After a couple of days of frequent feedings, your milk supply will have increased to meet your infant's needs. Remember to keep your fluid level up, too, because it takes fluid to make milk for your baby.

Occasionally, tension and stress may affect your milk production. At such times, a glass of beer (dark ale has Vitamin B) may help to relax you, facilitating the let-down reflex. Your relaxation techniques, also, can be valuable when you breastfeed.

Still Going . . .

Enjoy the time you spend nursing your baby. Do not waste this time worrying about housework or other problems. A new baby always requires some adjustment of your schedule. You may need to re-evaluate your priorities. Try to organize your time to make things easier for yourself. Do not plan to clean thoroughly, but content yourself with straightening up superficially. Housework and jobs will always be there, but your baby is little for such a short time. Relax, and enjoy his babyhood.

Even when the nursing relationship is good, there are times when the mother feels used and abused. The demands of nursing may leave you little time for yourself. While you are nursing your baby, you must remember that you are still a woman and a wife. Make time to fulfill your own needs and those of your husband. You were a person first, then a wife, then a mother. These other roles will exist after your children are grown and have left home. Do not let yourself become so thoroughly absorbed in motherhood that you let your other relationships suffer. Spend time on yourself. Take a long luxurious bath or shower, follow it with a careful make-up application, and dress yourself in something especially attractive. If your breasts are not too large, you can replace your nursing bra with a low-cut, lacy bra that has good support. Just pull the cup down to nurse; then, after the baby is done, replace the cup. Find someone you trust to care for your baby while you get away for a while, either alone or with your husband. Sometimes, this will be all that you need. Fathers should understand how demanding the role of motherhood is, especially when the baby is very young.

Gone . . .

The end of nursing is called **weaning**. This process can be initiated by the baby or the mother. Your baby may gradually lose interest in nursing as he becomes more active and begins to eat and drink with the rest of the family. Some babies become fascinated with doing things for themselves at about nine months of age, and want to do what everyone else does—drink from a cup. As your baby becomes more interested in his surroundings and better able to control some of them, he may not want to spend as much time nursing. He will prefer to be up and about. This may be a sad time for you as you see your tiny one growing up, but it will also be exciting.

Your baby may gradually decrease the nursing time, until he nurses only when he is hurt and wants comfort or before going to sleep.

At some point you may feel that the disadvantages of nursing have come to outweigh the advantages, and may decide to stop nursing before your baby initiates weaning. Do not feel guilty. If you are unhappy, your baby will sense this and be unhappy too. Good mothering involves recognizing the needs of all the family members and reacting appropriately. You are one of these members. If you decide to wean your baby, it is best to skip one feeding a day until the baby is no longer nursing. Usually, a feeding during the day is easier to omit than the feedings before bedtime or in the early morning. You will experience less engorgement and discomfort if you wean gradually.

Nursing is a very intense personal relationship and is different for each person. Whatever makes you feel comfortable will be right for you and your family.

During your nursing experience you may have many questions. This chapter cannot possibly answer all of them. Organizations exist that educate and support the nursing mother. The most well-known one is La Leche League. This international organization may have a chapter in your area. Your health care provider can help you to contact these organizations. Please call them if you have any problems, as they are the real authorities in the field, and are eager to help you.

BOTTLE FEEDING

You have read about breastfeeding, its advantages and disadvantages. Now let us consider the advantages and disadvantages of bottle feeding an infant. Every positive aspect of breastfeeding has its negative counterpart in bottle feeding, and vice versa. For example, a disadvantage of breastfeeding is that only the mother can feed the baby, whereas anyone can bottle feed a baby. Reread the section on the disadvantages of breastfeeding. These are the advantages of bottle feeding. The situation in your home and family will help determine which method of infant feeding you choose.

There is some controversy over the necessity of sterilizing bottles, the need to warm the milk before feeding, and the amount of formula the baby should be fed. Most women rely on the recommendations of their physicians. If you are going to use sterile bottles, you can either sterilize them yourself, or use pre-sterilized disposable units. Your decision about what brand of formula to use will probably be influenced by your doctor. This may change as you evaluate your baby's response to the formula.

There are some concerns that affect all mothers, regardless of the method of feeding. These include the quantity of food the baby takes and the quality of his stool. The breastfeeding mother wonders if he is getting enough, and the bottle-feeding mother wonders if he is getting enough or too much. Your doctor will recommend how many ounces of formula you should feed your baby and how often you should feed him. You may wonder if this is the right amount when your baby appears frequently fussy, or when he wakes too early and cries for his bottle. You will also feel concerned if he appears to be gaining too much or too little weight. You may need to experiment a little. If your child appears to be gaining too much weight, try a pacifier to see if that satisfies him. Many babies need to suck frequently. Some mothers reject the idea of a pacifier. They visualize how he will look in kindergarten and what the other kids will say if he refuses to give it up. Most children readily give the pacifier up when they no longer want to suck as much.

The frequency of the infant's bowel movements (0–10 a day) is not as important as the consistency of the stools. If they are soft, you needn't worry. If the stools are hard, rock-like pellets that are difficult for the baby to pass, your doctor may suggest changing formula if the baby is bottle-fed. Propping the baby in an infant seat will enable gravity to help the process of elimination.

INTRODUCING SOLIDS

A frequent concern of parents is when and how to add solid foods to the baby's diet. The American Academy of Pediatrics recommends that the infant be given only breast milk or formula for the first four to six months of life. He does not need juice, water, nor any solids until then, and his system is not sufficiently mature before that time to benefit from solid foods. In addition, the chances of inducing food allergies are greatest during the first few months of life.

After six months you can gradually add solids, one at a time. Feed each new food to your baby for one week, being sure to give him that food every day during that week. This will enable you to easily identify food allergies. Your baby can probably begin eating foods from your table, as long as you do not oversalt the food. A good first food is mashed ripe banana. If he likes the mashed banana, wait one week before adding meat or boiled egg yolks (not whites). These are good sources of iron. Then follow with whole grain cereal without added sweetener, and whole wheat bread cut into finger-sized pieces. Potatoes, fruits, and finally vegetables can then be introduced. Avoid giving him egg whites and whole milk until he is about one year old to avoid food allergies. Introduce the solids gradually—soon your baby will be eating the same foods the rest of the family eats.

All food should be mashed and moistened with water, breast milk, or formula, until it reaches a consistency that is appropriate for the baby's age. Gradually moisten it less, until it approaches the consistency of the food that you feed the rest of the family. When you prepare the baby's food, make a larger amount than needed and fill an ice cube tray with the extra meat or vegetables. When frozen, remove the cubes and place them in plastic freezer bags. You can then remove as many cubes as you feel are necessary to heat for a meal when the time comes. Table food mashed to the proper consistency for your baby is fine, as long as it is not highly salted, sweetened, or spiced. When the family is eating highly-seasoned foods, the frozen cubes will come in handy.

Your baby will probably be able to feed himself most of the time. Remember, though, that he will be slower and more messy than you are. Try not to force the baby to eat something he does not want. If your baby does not like a certain food, stop offering it to him, and reintroduce the food later.

During your baby's first year of life, you will be setting his pattern of food preferences. Avoid offering him foods with little or no nutritional value. Remember that processed food has lost much of its nutrients. Offer instead a variety of wholesome, natural foods to all the members of your family, including the baby. That way, everyone will benefit.

Chapter Seven
Here We Go Again: Welcoming More Children Into Your Family

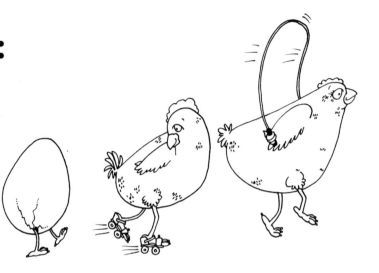

In our culture, it is often assumed that once you have experienced pregnancy and childbirth, there will not be much more to learn during the following pregnancies. Friends, relatives, and even your husband may not be as excited or as concerned when you discover your second pregnancy. You may enter into it with the confidence of one who is travelling down a well-known path, sure of your ability to anticipate and identify each step along the way. This is often the case. You now have successfully borne a child and are parenting with some confidence. You may be less worried about how the new baby should be fed, how he should be bathed, and how soon you should take him shopping with you.

However, like snowflakes, no two pregnancies are alike. If you expect each pregnancy to follow the pattern of the first experience, you may be suddenly surprised. You would never expect all of your children to be identical in appearance, temperament, or intelligence. In the same way, it is important for you to realize that each pregnancy and birth will be just as unique and special as each newborn infant.

THE PHYSICAL ASPECTS OF PREGNANCY

As your pregnancy progresses, you may notice that your physical sensations are different from those of your first pregnancy. Many women find that the uterus enlarges more quickly (so that the need to dig out your maternity clothes may come sooner than you had hoped!). You may also feel the baby move much earlier in your pregnancy. Do you remember feeling "butterflies" in your uterus during your first pregnancy? You were never sure whether it was intestinal gas or the movements of your baby. It took a while for you to be sure of what you felt. This time you will identify your baby's movements with expertise, and enjoy his company.

Besides taking care of yourself during the progressing pregnancy, you will now also be caring for your other children as well as performing household chores and, perhaps, doing outside work. Many women find themselves more fatigued during this later pregnancy, so you may have to re-evaluate your priorities in order to get some needed rest. (It's a real trick to sneak in a nap when your toddler is splashing in the toilet!)

As your pregnancy continues, you may feel much "bigger" than you remember feeling during previous experiences. Your baby may feel heavier to carry. Along with these sensations, many women have more backaches, sharp pains, and dull aches in the groin. The abdominal muscles may not support the uterus as well as they did in your first pregnancy. Consequently, the growing uterus may tilt forward, placing more pressure on the area of the pubic bone. Your uterus may not be very different in size, but you will be carrying it differently than before. As the uterus leans forward, stress is added to the uterine ligaments that are attached in the small of your back, causing a backache. You will need to watch your posture and how you move about. Carrying toddlers and picking up small toys (or even large socks) can put more strain on back muscles and ligaments if not done properly.

You may experience more Braxton-Hicks contractions than before. During your first pregnancy you may not have realized that you were experiencing contractions until your childbirth instructor identified them for you. Now you may feel them early in your pregnancy and find that they are stronger and come more frequently as the pregnancy progresses. Many women experience times of "false labor" during which the contractions continue for some time before tapering off. This can get frustrating, since it will have you sitting on the edge of your chair during the last few weeks, thinking the birth will be earlier than expected! Yet, you may feel silly leaving the hospital after a false alarm. (After all, others might think that since you've done this before, you should know when labor begins!) The Braxton-Hicks contractions can get quite strong, and may be hard to distinguish from early labor contractions.

You may also find that this baby will not engage (drop) before labor begins. In the first pregnancy, the baby usually descends into the pelvis sometime before labor contractions. The next baby may not move deep into the pelvis until sometime during labor or delivery.

THE EMOTIONAL ASPECTS OF PREGNANCY

After discovering your pregnancy, you may be surprised by the reactions of others to your good news. Friends and relatives may not be as interested or excited as they were when you had your first baby. In fact, with another child on the way, you may hear differing opinions of how you should have planned your family. In our society, a first-born child is well accepted by almost everyone, whether or not that pregnancy was planned. You are moved through rituals designed to welcome you into the world of parenting: the purchase of a new wardrobe, baby showers, and childbirth classes.

During your second pregnancy, you may find less interest from others, except for their excitement over your chance to have a baby of the opposite sex (whether or not you care). During your third pregnancy, you may encounter questioning looks, unless you have two children of the same sex; then it will be considered all right to try again for that opposite sex. During a fourth pregnancy, few people know what to say. Reactions range from congratulations to condolences. You may get unwanted advice and comments: concern over your health and sanity, uneasiness about your financial ability to care for your family, thoughts about the needs of your other children, and distress over your continuing fertility in the future ("What are you going to *do* after the baby is born?"). Once into your fifth pregnancy, any comments or suggestions may stop, for you are surely exceptional! Our society has certain ideas about family size, and few people keep their opinions to themselves.

Despite what others may think, you and your husband may be thrilled by the addition of more children to your family. You may have wonderful memories of your children as infants and delight in watching your children develop and grow. You have gained skills and confidence in parenting, and may be eager to enjoy another child. Some women are distressed by their husband's reaction to another pregnancy. Your husband may be unsure of his feelings. As a mother, you personally experience the differences between pregnancies, and can more easily identify the different personalities of the babies you carry. You may feel some resentment if your husband appears less excited or interested in sharing this pregnancy, and worry that this lack of interest will carry into his feelings for your child.

You should also seriously consider your own feelings about this pregnancy. With your first baby, the excitement, support, and care you received from others may have eased you through any periods of ambivalence. During this pregnancy, however, you will probably receive less attention and support. Therefore, if you are not sure of your feelings about the pregnancy, you may experience greater frustration and anxiety than you did during your previous pregnancy. Some women feel guilty over the fact that they are not enjoying this pregnancy as they enjoyed others, that these feelings may somehow affect their baby, and that they will not be able to spend more time with their other children before adding another baby to the family. They may worry also about their ability to love the coming child.

The rituals of baby showers and gifts surrounding first pregnancies are not just ways of collecting possessions. They are ways for those who care for you to express their support and encouragement of your decision to have this child. Unfortunately, these traditions are not always carried on as you welcome more children into your family.

CHILDBIRTH

After having had one memorable birth, you may be looking forward to another exhilarating labor. Having borne children before, you may be eagerly anticipating childbirth with confidence and, perhaps, expectations of a job well done. You may feel comfortable regarding labor, and secure about issues that previously frightened you.

While some women eagerly anticipate the vigorous activity and accomplishment of labor and birth, others find that they are more fearful of the coming labor. Friends and relatives may never acknowledge this fear, thinking that having once experienced childbirth, the mother should easily give birth again. The mother may feel isolated and foolish about her fear and wish that she could postpone labor or, perhaps, eliminate it altogether.

If your previous labor was difficult, you may be worried about handling a similar experience. Even if your past labor was fairly smooth, you might be apprehensive that this birth could become more difficult. Taking time to prepare for the birth may help give you the confidence you need. Attending refresher classes and discovering that other women share these feelings also may help.

After a review of preparation techniques, you may be ready for birth. Although each labor is unique, many women expect future births to be similar to previous ones. This labor, however, may start in a different way, and may be shorter. (But don't expect each successive birth to take less and less time until there is no labor at all!) Since the cervix has effaced and dilated before, the effacement will occur more easily. Since the tissues of the birth canal have bloomed before, the birth of your baby, also, may take place quickly. Instead of a gradual build-up of pressure as you push the baby down, your breath may be taken away as the baby quickly appears at the vaginal opening. Other variations, including the position of the baby, the length of time between births, and the size of the baby can influence how greatly this birth differs from past births.

It is important to be aware of the variables rather than to sit back, smugly ready to slip into the labor patterns you previously established. Well before your due date, you should review the choices available to you at your hospital or birth center (e.g., rooming-in, siblings at birth, sibling visitation, etc.). Many changes may have taken place, so you'll want to plan your birth with these new alternatives in mind.

The immediate recovery time may be exhilarating. There will be a need to watch the uterus to make sure that it contracts firmly to prevent any excessive bleeding. It may not contract as spontaneously as it did after your previous birth. Nursing your baby will promote uterine contractions; if not, Pitocin may be administered. During the first few days after birth, you may experience "afterpains." These are contractions that begin to reduce the uterus to its nonpregnant size and weight. Although these contractions are seldom noticed after a first birth, they may be very apparent after successive births, especially while breastfeeding.

If you give birth in a hospital, you may find that you want to extend your postpartum stay indefinitely! You may feel much better than you anticipated, and may wish to have your husband and other children there with you. You may not feel ready to return to your old routine. However, relatives, your husband, or even you may expect that, once home again, you will be able to quickly resume your chores. Be sure to allow yourself a period of recovery, with special privileges, adequate rest, and time to get acquainted with your new infant without too much interference.

You may find that tending your infant comes easily. The skills and confidence you gathered in the past may enable you to streamline your infant care schedule. You may even find that the task of adding another child's care to your family's routine is less difficult than you expected.

Many of the questions and concerns you had after your first baby have already been answered. At the same time, you may find that caring for more children forces you to change your priorities. There will be more chores to handle and less time in which they must be accomplished. Sharing these tasks with your husband and your other children can help. You might begin handling housework with a quick once-over and a promise to attend to it fully at another time. The time you spend with your children and husband is what your family will remember—not cobwebs and messy closets.

SIBLINGS

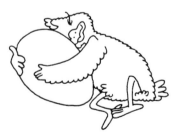

When you bring your new baby home, your older child will experience a wide range of emotions. This will be a time of sadness, because your child's relationship with you will never be the same, and a time of pleasant expectation, because, in time, he will have the companionship of a sibling. Every child wants the exclusive attention of his parents. Whenever this is threatened, he will experience a sense of loss and fear. Your child may wonder how your relationship will change. How can you love another? Why doesn't he satisfy you? Why do you want another? Your child needs your reassurance that your love will always be there—that your love for him is special, and will not be given to another child.

If this is your second child, you and your husband, also, may be concerned about how your relationship with another child will affect your first-born. Perhaps your first child is still young. You may feel that you are not going to be able to give him the attention that he needs, now that you will be caring for an infant. Maybe your first-born is older, and you are concerned about how he will feel about sharing your attention. You may even fear that you will be taking love away from your first-born to love another child. Be assured that just as each child is unique, so will be your love for each one. Your love will not be divided among your children, but will grow and blossom.

A sudden leap in development will occur as your child's role and position in your family changes. There will be new and different privileges, as well as new responsibilities. The coming of a baby is a part of growing up. Sibling relationships provide an opportunity to become aware of the rights of others. With brothers and sisters, your child will continue to learn how to give and receive love, work out differences, and share common feelings. Parents often expect rivalry with the introduction of a baby, and may overlook the bond of affection developing between their children. Don't underestimate your child's understanding. The baby will mean as much to him as to you. Be aware of the intensity of his feelings. You are all having this baby.

Just how your child reacts will depend on several factors. You might try to recall your response to a new brother or sister in order to understand your child's thoughts. No matter what the age of your child, during your pregnancy it will be obvious to him that you are different. Your body will change, you will tire easily, and your moods will shift. Because of your child's observations, you may see reactions before the baby arrives. When the baby becomes part of your family, it will be apparent to your child that the baby's care takes a great deal of time. He will attempt to remain the center of your attention. His reactions will sometimes be easy to see, and will sometimes be rather subtle.

Regressive Behavior

Some children return to infantile forms of behavior, trying to become the baby their parents want. They may ask for pacifiers again, or begin sucking a thumb more often than usual. They may want to drink out of a bottle, or show interest in nursing. Other children use baby talk, crawl, or ask to be fed by their parents. Many stay close to their mother, not wanting to be separated from her. Nightmares and sleeping disturbances such as bedwetting may occur, especially if the child has recently changed beds or been moved into a different room. If the baby sleeps in the parents' bedroom, the older child may want to sleep there too. Parents often anticipate some regression with toilet training, but this is not common, and seems to happen only when other stresses surround the birth (such as starting school or moving into a new house).

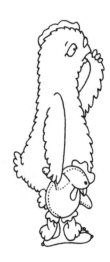

Aggressive Behavior

If your child is talking, he may verbally express his hostility: "Take the baby back to the hospital now," "Flush the baby down the toilet," or "Put the baby in the garbage can . . . and don't forget to put the lid on!" Remember that he is concerned about his changing relationship with you, and wants your attention first. He is not reacting to the baby as much as he is to having less time with you.

Some children try to hurt the baby by hitting or biting. You can see the anger they have for this "intruder." Of course, you cannot allow your children to hurt the baby. Other children are overly affectionate—almost too loving—and you might find them hugging the baby too hard or playing a bit rough. Encourage your child to defuse these hostile feelings. Reading children's books that describe these emotions may help, and vigorous outdoor activity can aid him in venting his feelings. His emotions may be hard for him to sort out. He really loves his sibling, but is angry about how he has disrupted his life. This child needs your guidance and your reassurance that his feelings are okay, that you understand, and that you will always love him.

Growing Up

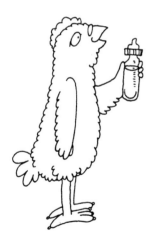

Just as this is a time of change, so is it a time of growth. Your child will be proud to be a big brother or big sister. Now may be the time he gives up baby ways. He may no longer want his bottle, pacifier, or special blanket. This may be the time he starts to use the toilet like Mom and Dad. He may begin to develop concern for others and to learn to become independent in his play and personal care. Since you will not have as much time to spend with him, he may develop a close relationship with someone near to him, such as his grandparents or baby sitters. Some children handle the stress they feel by sharing it with an imaginary companion.

You can ease your older child's adjustment in several ways. Preparing for the baby's birth is essential. Share your pregnancy with him. Some couples break the news as soon as the pregnancy is confirmed. Others wait until early in the second trimester, as the mother's appearance begins to change and fetal movement becomes apparent. Don't let your child learn of your pregnancy from someone else.

Be sensitive to your child's age and personality. Too much information is confusing for smaller children, and too little information is unsatisfying for older ones. Answer your child's questions honestly. Children are usually curious about how the baby grows and how he will get out. The fantasies children have about the birth process may be frightening. (Children often imagine the baby being born through the mother's navel or through her mouth.) Books that display photographs of early uterine development and birth may be helpful. As the baby grows, your child might want to feel him moving or kicking.

Take time to discuss how you will care for your baby, and be sure to be realistic in your description. Your children may become friends in the years to come, but your child might expect the baby to be a playmate at birth. Visiting friends who have infants will reinforce your description of what a newborn is really like. Try to visit more than one baby, or your child may be surprised if his baby isn't exactly the same as the one he saw. Providing your child with a doll or small pet can help to teach him ways of handling things gently and with care. You might bring him along for your prenatal visits. Most attendants will be willing to let your child listen to the baby's heartbeat and to describe the baby's position.

Include your child in your preparations. Shopping for baby clothes and accessories and decorating the baby's room or corner can be fun to do together. When you unpack clothes and blankets, it will be a good time to reminisce about your older child's birth and infancy.

Your feelings about the baby will be apparent to your child, even before the birth. Try to include him in your discussions, and don't hide your feelings of excitement or apprehension. Perhaps you should consider your feelings at this point. What concerns do you have about bringing a baby into your family? How do you expect your child will react? How about your spouse?

Explain the arrangements for the birth—where you will be and who will be with him. Try not to disrupt your child's routine. If possible, let him remain at home during your hospital stay. Be sure to have someone he knows and trusts care for him. You might leave some personal items at home—perhaps a purse, your keys, or an eyeglass case—so that your child will be reassured that you will soon be home. Take advantage of the sibling classes or children's hospital tours in your area. If your child visits the hospital, he will have a better idea of where you are when the baby is being born, as the hospital will have become a real part of his world. This will comfort him.

Sibling Visitation

Many hospitals allow sibling visitation during the mother's hospital stay. It is important for your child, regardless of his age, to visit his mother. It may be fun for him to see and perhaps hold the baby. More crucial, however, is his visit with you. He needs to see that you and the baby are well, and that you miss him. This is another way to include him in the excitement

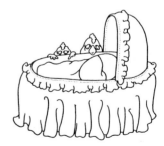

surrounding birth. He knows that many friends visit his mother, and he may feel proud and grown-up to be one of her visitors. This is also a way for your child to ask questions and accept the birth experience before you come home, so that your homecoming will be more casual and pleasant. Be aware that this can become a bittersweet moment. Spending time together will be delightful, but when he goes home it may bring tears for all of you. Your child might not understand that you cannot go with him. However, don't let this discourage you from bringing your child to the hospital. It is important that he spend time with you. Phone calls and notes cannot replace a visit with you. You might consider an early discharge from the hospital if you are confident of having help at home.

Much gift giving usually surrounds the birth. Your child might wish to choose a gift to bring the baby when he visits the hospital. Sometimes, there is a gift from the baby to his older brother or sister, and when friends and relatives bring presents for the baby and mother, they may want to bring a small gift for the older child. The really special present, however, is the one that the child brings to his mother. He knows others are bringing gifts, and he wants to be included. Follow your family traditions.

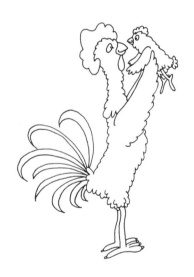

Other Aspects of Sibling Adjustment

As your family settles in after birth, you will want to tell your child of the pride you feel in his growth and his acceptance of new responsibilities. Include him in the care of your baby, if he likes. He may be delighted to fetch diapers or to talk to the baby as you watch nearby. Let your child know that you love him uniquely. You can't love your children equally, so don't try to. Your love for each child will be special, and will grow and develop as they do. Avoid making comparisons. Take time to spend with your child. The time you spend listening to him is more important than field trips or after-school activities.

With the birth of another baby, the father may become more involved with the older child. This increased attention from his father during pregnancy, at birth when his mother is in the hospital, and when the family is settling in at home can significantly diminish negative sibling reactions.

When special problems occur with the newborn, such as an illness or death, your child will be aware that something is wrong. Try to explain the situation to him, keeping his age and personality in mind. Some parents transfer the child's care to a friend or relative to protect him from sadness. This may not be in your child's best interests. Not only will he know that something is wrong, but he may be distressed by his separation from you. His fantasies of what is happening may be more difficult to handle than the truth. He may need your reassurance that he is not the cause of the problem, and that this same problem will not happen to him.

Share your feelings with him. Your child is better able to handle and accept your feelings of anxiety, sadness, and grief than he is able to suffer the withdrawal of parents who hide their true emotions. Include your child in the funeral proceedings. His exclusion may indicate to him that you are unaware of his feeling of sadness over the loss of the baby, or that death is secret and frightening. This may be an experience that you can best handle as a family.

You cannot prevent your child from experiencing changes when another baby is born, nor should you want to. This is a special time for him. Sometimes he may become frustrated. At other times he may wish life to be as it was before the pregnancy. It is your relationship with him that is most important. He needs to be assured of your continued love and approval. It is a time for him to grow and learn to become independent.

With each additional pregnancy you will discover how unique every child is, even before that child's birth. With each child, as you become more confident in your parenting, you will become less concerned about the chores of child rearing and more involved in the development of your family bond. So take time to enjoy! Enjoy yourself, enjoy your spouse, and enjoy all your children!

Recommended Reading

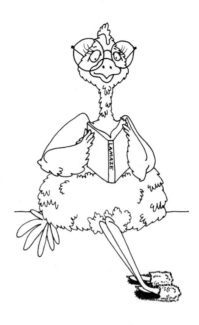

Berezin, Nancy. *The Gentle Birth Book*. New York: Simon and Schuster, Inc., 1980.

Bing, Elisabeth, ed. *The Adventure of Birth*. New York: Simon and Schuster, Inc., 1970.

Bing, Elisabeth. *Six Practical Lessons for an Easier Childbirth*. New York: Grosset and Dunlap, Inc., 1967.

Bing, Elisabeth, and Colman, Libby. *Making Love During Pregnancy*. New York: Bantam Books, Inc., 1977.

Bing, Elisabeth, and Karmel, Marjorie. *A Practical Training Course for the Psychoprophylactic Method of Childbirth*. New York: ASPO, 1960.

Boston Women's Health Book Collective. *Our Bodies, Ourselves*. New York: Simon and Schuster, Inc., 1973.

Brewer, Gail, ed. *The Pregnancy After 30 Workbook*. Emmaus, Pennsylvania: Rodale Press, Inc., 1978.

Brewer, Gail Sforza, and Brewer, Tom. *What Every Pregnant Woman Should Know: The Truth About Diet and Drugs During Pregnancy*. New York: Random House, Inc., 1977.

Brinkley, Ginny; Goldberg, Linda; and Kukar, Janet. *Your Child's First Journey: A Guide to Prepared Birth From Pregnancy to Parenthood.* Wayne, New Jersey: Avery Publishing Group, Inc., 1982.

Chabon, Irwin. *Awake and Aware.* New York: Dell Publishing Co., Inc., 1966.

Dick-Read, Grantly. *Childbirth Without Fear.* 2nd ed. New York: Harper and Row Publishers, Inc., 1953.

Downing, George, and Rush, Anne Kent. *The Massage Book.* New York: Random House, Inc., and California: Bookworks, 1972.

Ewy, Donna, and Ewy, Rodger. *Preparation for Childbirth.* Boulder, Colorado: Pruett Publishing Co., 1972.

Hazell, Lester Dessez. *Commonsense Childbirth.* New York: Putnam, 1969.

Karmel, Marjorie. *Thank You, Dr. Lamaze.* New York: Doubleday and Co., Inc., 1965.

Kitzinger, Sheila. *The Experience of Childbirth.* New York: Taplinger Publishing Co., Inc., 1974.

Kitzinger, Sheila. *Giving Birth.* New York: Taplinger Publishing Co., Inc., 1971.

La Leche League International. *The Womanly Art of Breastfeeding.* New York: The New American Library, Inc., 1984.

Lamaze, Fernand. *Painless Childbirth: The Lamaze Method.* New York: Henry Regnery Co., 1970.

Lauwers, Judith; Woessner, Candace; CEA of Greater Philadelphia. *Counseling the Nursing Mother: A Reference Handbook for Health Care Providers and Lay Counselors.* Wayne, New Jersey: Avery Publishing Group, Inc., 1983.

Leboyer, Frederick. *Birth Without Violence.* New York: Alfred A. Knopf, Inc., 1976.

Lexington Association for Parent Education. *Your Child's Birth: A Comprehensive Guide for Pregnancy, Birth, and Postpartum.* Wayne, New Jersey: Avery Publishing Group, Inc., 1983.

Maternity Center Association. *A Baby is Born.* New York: Grosset and Dunlap, Inc., 1965.

Maternity Center Association. *Guide for Expectant Parents.* New York: Grosset and Dunlap, Inc., 1954.

Montagu, Ashley. *Life Before Birth.* New York: The New American Library, Inc., 1965.

Nilsson, Lennart. *A Child is Born.* New York: Delacorte Press, 1977.

Noble, Elizabeth. *Essential Exercises for the Childbearing Year.* Boston: Houghton Mifflin Co., 1982.

Nursing Mothers' Council of the Boston Association for Childbirth Education. *Breast-Feeding Your Baby.* 2nd ed. Wayne, New Jersey: Avery Publishing Group, Inc., 1981.

Pryor, Karen. *Nursing Your Baby*. New York: Harper and Row Publishers, Inc., 1973.

Rush, Anne Kent. *Getting Clear*. New York: Random House, Inc., 1973.

Seidman, Theodore, and Albert, Marvin. *Becoming a Mother*. Greenwich, Connecticut: Lawcett Publications, Inc., 1956.

Tanger, Deborah, and Block, Jean Libman. *Why Natural Childbirth?* New York: Doubleday and Co., Inc., 1972.

Vellay, Pierre. *Childbirth Without Pain*. Translated by Denise Lloyd. New York: E.P. Dutton, Inc., 1959.

Wilson, Christine, and Hovey, Wendy. *Cesarean Childbirth: A Handbook for Parents*. Ann Arbor, Michigan: Wilson and Hovey, 1977.

Wright, Erna. *The New Childbirth*. New York: Hart Publishing Co., 1967.

Glossary

abruptio placentae. Premature separation of normally implanted placenta.

afterbirth. The discharge of placenta and membranes that passes out of the uterus during the third stage of labor.

afterpains. The contractions of the uterus that follow birth.

amnihook. An obstetrical instrument used to rupture the amniotic sac, either to permit the insertion of a fetal monitor probe or to induce or augment labor.

amniocentesis. The procedure of passing a needle through the abdominal wall to withdraw fluid from the amniotic sac. The fluid can then be tested to determine fetal maturity, the sex of the baby, antibody formation, or the presence or absence of many congenital abnormalities.

amniotic sac (bag of waters). The membranous sac containing the amniotic fluid and the fetus. The amniotic fluid absorbs shock and provides the fetus with an environment of constant pressure and temperature.

analgesics. Drugs used to relieve pain without causing unconsciousness.

anesthetics. Drugs used to induce a loss of

sensation, with or without a loss of consciousness.

areola. The ring of pigment surrounding the nipple.

back labor. Labor experienced in the lower back, buttocks, and thighs, occurring either during contractions or continuously. Back labor is caused by the position of the baby, the anatomy of the mother, or other factors. Relief measures include position changes, counterpressure, and massage.

bloody show. The loss of the mucous plug, occurring either weeks or days before labor begins or during labor. This "show" consists of a thick, jelly-like substance, and may be tinged with blood.

bonding. The establishment of the mother/ child/father relationship immediately following birth.

Braxton-Hicks contractions. Sometimes called false labor contractions, these intermittent contractions occur periodically throughout pregnancy as the uterus prepares for labor.

breech position. The fetal birth position in which the baby's buttocks or feet are presenting first.

centimeter (cm). The unit of measure used to describe the progress of cervical dilation. 1 cm is equal to .3937 inches.

cephalopelvic disproportion. A condition in which the baby's head is too large to fit through the mother's pelvis. Usually, this condition necessitates cesarean delivery.

cervix. The neck-like, narrow end of the uterus that opens into the vagina.

cesarean birth. The surgical removal of the baby through incisions made in the uterine and abdominal walls.

circumcision. The surgical removal of the foreskin of the penis.

colostrum. An early form of breastmilk, colostrum is the first substance a breast-fed baby receives. It is uniquely suited for the newborn.

contractions. The involuntary tightening and shortening of the uterine muscles during labor, causing cervical effacement and dilation and facilitating the baby's descent.

crowning. The appearance of the presenting part of the baby—usually the head—at the vaginal opening.

dilation. The gradual opening of the cervix to permit the baby to pass out of the uterus. The degree of dilation is expressed in centimeters, and dilation is said to be complete at 10 centimeters.

edema. An excessive accumulation of fluid in the body tissues.

effacement. The thinning and shortening of the cervix. Effacement is expressed in terms of percentage.

effleurage. The gentle stroking of the lower abdomen used during labor to soothe and relax the mother's abdominal muscles.

enema. The injection of a solution (usually soap and water) into the rectum to clean out the bowel in preparation for labor and birth.

engagement. The securing of the baby's presenting part into the opening (inlet) of the pelvic cavity.

engorgement. A painful swelling of the tissues of the breast caused by an increased blood supply and the accumulation of milk.

episiotomy. The incision made into the perineum prior to delivery, enlarging the vaginal outlet to prevent laceration or to facilitate delivery.

estriol determination test. The prenatal evaluation of the mother's estriol level for the purpose of assessing placental function and fetal well-being.

false labor. Contractions strong enough to be interpreted as true labor, but having no dilating effect on the cervix.

fetal distress. A condition in which the baby shows signs of oxygen deprivation.

fetal monitor. A machine used to detect and record labor contractions and the fetal heart rate.

fetus. The term used to refer to the baby from the eighth week after conception until birth.

forceps. A tong-like obstetrical instrument used to correct the baby's position or to ease his passage out of the birth canal.

hemorrhoids. Varicose veins that develop in the rectum.

hypertension. High blood pressure.

hyperventilation. A condition caused by the exhalation of too much carbon dioxide and characterized by dizziness, tingling hands and feet, and muscle spasms. Hyperventilation can be corrected by breathing into cupped hands or a paper bag.

hypotension. Blood pressure that is lower than normal.

induction. The initiation of labor by medication or the artificial rupture of the amniotic sac.

intravenous (IV) fluid. A sterile fluid administered via a needle that is inserted into a vein in the mother's forearm. The IV drip is used to provide nutrition, hydration, or medication.

in utero. Within the uterus.

involution. The return of the female reproductive organs to a nonpregnant state after delivery, taking approximately six weeks.

Kegel exercise. An exercise devised by Dr. Arnold Kegel to strengthen the muscles of the pelvic floor.

Leboyer birth. Named after Frederick Leboyer, this is a quiet, peaceful form of delivery that is designed to reduce the trauma of birth.

let-down reflex. The pattern of stimulation, hormonal release, and resultant muscle contractions that forces milk into the ducts leading to the areola and nipple area of the breast. Through this process, milk is made available to the baby during breastfeeding.

lochia. The discharge of blood, mucus, and tissue from the uterus after birth. This may continue for two to four weeks.

molding. The shaping of the baby's head to conform to the contours of the birth canal.

mucous plug. The plug of heavy mucus that blocks the cervical canal during pregnancy, preventing foreign matter from entering the uterus.

multipara. A woman who has given birth to more than one child.

Non-Stress Test (NST). A prenatal test performed with the aid of the external fetal monitor to assess the baby's reactions to his own movements, and thus evaluate fetal well-being.

oxytocin. The hormone that stimulates uterine contractions and the let-down reflex.

Oxytocin Challenge Test (OCT) or Stress Test. A prenatal test performed with the aid of the external fetal monitor to assess the baby's response to drug-induced contractions, and thus evaluate fetal well-being.

pelvic floor. The hammock-like structure, composed of ligaments and muscles, that supports the reproductive organs.

perineum. The external tissues surrounding the anus and the vagina.

Pitocin. The synthetic form of the hormone oxytocin.

placenta. The vascular structure developed during pregnancy that allows for the exchange of nutrients and fetal waste.

placenta previa. An abnormal implantation of the placenta, partially or completely blocking the cervical opening.

posterior position. A fetal birth position in which the back of the baby's head is against the mother's spine.

postpartum period. The first six weeks following childbirth.

prep. The shaving or clipping of the pubic hair in preparation for birth.

presentation. The position of the baby in the

uterus. The presenting part of the baby is that part which is closest to the cervix.

primigravida. A woman who is pregnant for the first time.

primipara. A woman who is pregnant for the first time or has borne just one child.

psychoprophylaxis. Literally meaning "mind prevention," this term describes the Lamaze technique of childbirth preparation, which prevents pain in labor by conditioning the mind to react to specific stimuli in specific ways.

rooming-in. An arrangement that enables mother and baby to stay in the same hospital room for an extended period of time.

rooting reflex. The newborn instinct that causes the infant to turn toward a touch on the cheek or mouth.

station. The location of the presenting part of the baby in relation to the ischial spines of the mother's pelvis. Negative stations $(-1, -2, -3)$ are successively higher; the zero station is level with the spines, and indicates engagement; positive stations $(+1, +2, +3)$ are successively lower and closer to the vaginal opening.

ultrasound scan. A procedure that directs sound waves towards the expectant mother's abdomen and transmits an image of the baby and the placenta onto a screen. Ultrasound may be used to determine the location, size, and number of babies *in utero*; to detect placenta previa; or to determine the due date.

umbilical cord. Composed of two arteries and one vein, this cord connects the unborn baby to the placenta, allowing the baby to receive nutrients and eliminate waste products.

uterus. Also called the womb, this is the organ of gestation.

vacuum extractor. An obstetrical instrument that uses suction to correct the baby's position or to ease the baby down the birth canal.

vagina. The curved, elastic canal that allows the baby to pass out of the uterus.

varicose veins. Enlarged veins, sometimes found in the legs, vulva (the external female reproductive organs), or rectum during pregnancy.

vernix. The white, cheese-like substance that protects the baby's skin *in utero*.

vertex position. The fetal birth position in which the head is the presenting part. This is the most common birth position.

Wharton's Jelly. The gelatin-like material that surrounds the umbilical cord.

Index

Childbirth Books From **Avery**

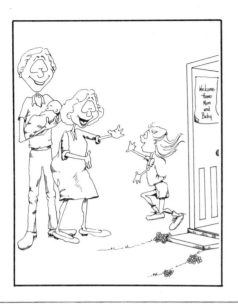

Our Family Grows
A Coloring & Activity Book
Renee Neri

Beautifully designed to prepare and involve the young child whose mother will soon be giving birth. Includes cut-outs, pictures for coloring, and creative activities for the sister or brother-to-be. Large type, simple instructions and amusing cartoons allow the child to have hours and hours of constructive fun. The time spent coloring, cutting, and drawing in *Our Family Grows* will enable the child to share the excitement and joy of having a baby.

$3.95

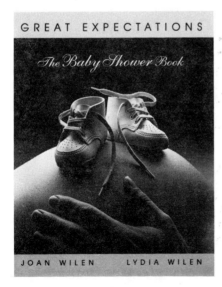

Great Expectations — A Baby Shower Book
Joan Wilen
Lydia Wilen

Here is a unique and novel way of recording the memories of your baby shower. *Great Expectations: A Baby Shower Book* invites family and friends to write down their predictions about the baby, give advice to the mother-to-be, and share their good wishes. Once the pages are filled, the book can be read to all, creating a fun and loving atmosphere. The perfect touch to a baby shower. Years from now, this treasured volume will be an affectionate memento of a meaningful time— your pregnancy. It also makes a great gift.

Just as every mother-to-be has great expectations, so should every baby shower have *Great Expectations*.

$6.95

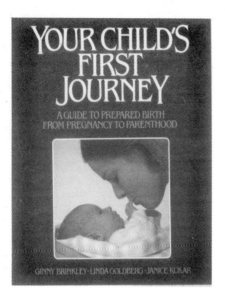

Your Child's First Journey
A Guide to Prepared Birth from Pregnancy to Parenthood
Ginny Brinkley   Linda Goldberg   Janice Kukar

Your Child's First Journey is a complete, fully illustrated book designed to accompany the expectant mother from the early months of pregnancy to the early months of parenthood. It is written with an emphasis on the emotional and physical benefits of family-centered care, and on the importance of being an educated consumer.

This comprehensive text encompasses all of the topics discussed in Early Pregnancy, Lamaze, Cesarean Preparation, and New Mothers' classes. Each section contains detailed coverage of an important aspect of pregnancy, birth, or infant care. Readers gain an awareness of current trends and controversies as they learn to make use of the most up-to-date childbirth techniques, and to become confident and capable parents.

$9.95